Simply
Well-Being

Your guide to
transforming your mental, physical
and spiritual well-being

Mary Parrish

Paperback: ISBN: 978-1-7392604-4-6
E-book ISBN: 978-1-7392604-2-2

For more information please visit
www.simply-well-being.com.

To my children.

Haydn, who has been a guiding force
from before he was born, who inspires me
to be a better version of myself.

Amanie, my greatest teacher,
who shows me daily that
there is so much more for me to learn.

I love you both.

Contents

Introduction

Welcome to my Simply Well-Being book. My aim with this book is to help you to stop and think about your own well-being, what it means to you and where you would like to make improvements or where you need help in order to live a fulfilled, happy and abundant life. I will provide some useful strategies and actions which can be incorporated into your daily routine to move you forward on your journey.

Why did I choose well-being? Throughout my life I have struggled with areas of mental well-being, physical well-being and spiritual well-being. I have found solutions and answers along the way, as well as learnt therapies, which have helped me to move forward and to heal myself. I would love to help you with whatever part of your well-being which needs focus. I will share with you parts of my journey, the steps I took and how I found solutions which have worked for me. I will also challenge you to find solutions which are right for you, as your journey will be different from mine.

You may choose to read the book chapter by chapter or you may dip in and out and read those topics which interest you the most. Whichever way you choose, I do hope that you are able to take away a few new methods to help you on your well-being journey. My wish is that there will be something which you have not thought of or considered before and which can help to improve your well-being from where you are today.

So, What Is Well-Being?

What does well-being mean for you?

I could ask a million people this question and would likely receive an array of thoughts and opinions on this topic ranging from fitness to food to feeling calm, well and happy. For me it is simple; well-being is to be healthy, happy and balanced.

We are all multi-dimensional beings which means that our well-being is also multi-faceted. It is not just about eating the right foods or thinking the right thoughts or exercising each day. To achieve overall, long lasting well-being we need to consider every aspect of our being, including our mental/psychological, physical and spiritual/emotional well-being. You may well be the biggest fitness fanatic on the planet but if your mental state is one of turmoil and stress then you will not be experiencing overall well-being. Similarly, if you have a Zen-like mind but only eat takeaways and junk food, then you are unlikely to be experiencing physical well-being or at least you won't be later in life if you continue down this track.

Achieving balance in all aspects of our multi-dimensional being is the Holy Grail. It is not about being perfect in all areas, but about finding your balance, what is right for you, what allows your energy and creativity to flow and what helps to keep you feeling calm, confident, healthy and happy.

How This Book Can Help You

During my journey I have read many books on health, well-being, mental health, spiritual healing and meditation. However, I haven't found one book which pulls all areas of well-being together in one place. To experience overall well-being, you can't just focus on one area. You are multi-faceted and therefore you need to consider mind, body and spirit. Consider the following questions. Do you:

- Frequently feel stressed or overwhelmed?
- Have trouble thinking straight or making decisions?
- Suffer with anxiety?
- Juggle so many activities but feel like you're not moving forward?
- Have trouble sleeping?
- Experience health concerns?
- Feel tired and fatigued?
- Struggle to lose weight?
- Experience headaches or migraines?
- Have sudden worries, anxiety or phobias which you never had before?
- Know you need to make a change but don't know where to start?

If you answered yes to any of the questions above, then this is the book for you. Come with me and let me help you on your journey.

I will discuss all elements of well-being, talk you through my journey and share with you the steps which I took to find solutions. I will also offer potential activities and strategies to help you discover what works for you. Your journey will be different from mine so I hope to provide you with some guidance and next steps which you can take on your well-being journey. Most sections include activities and exercises which you could add to your daily routine to help you to improve.

You may find that you are already taking care of one or two of these areas of well-being. Perhaps you have less interest or maybe less knowledge of the other area or areas which is where you need to improve your focus.

The strategies which I have included are not necessarily exclusive to that one section of well-being. The majority will bridge at least two areas, but I have included them in the section where I believe they primarily help. For example, exercise not only helps our physical well-being, but it also has a huge impact on our mood and mental wellness. Meditation not only helps our daily mental well-being but also our spiritual well-being too. See Appendix one for the strategy connections.

What Do I Mean By These Areas Of Well-Being?

Mental well-being – encompasses how you are thinking and feeling in your mind. This includes how you are feeling emotionally, how you react and handle situations in your day to day life such as stress and decision making, how you interact with others around you including your relationships, how you feel about yourself and how your mind feels on a daily basis. Are you calm, in control and feeling happy? Or are you living in a heightened state of sensitivity, stress, anxiety and feeling overwhelmed? I want you to remember that you are not a human doer, you are a human being and you need to re-learn to just be. It's OK just to be.

Physical well-being – encompasses how you are feeling within your body. Are you healthy and feeling well, energetic and full of life or are you regularly unwell with one complaint or another? Do you suffer with aches and pains or headaches?

Are you overweight? Are you unfit? Do you regularly feel tired and lethargic? All of these questions can help you to assess your overall physical well-being.

Spiritual well-being – encompasses how you are feeling about your life, purpose and connection with the outside world. Do you feel connected to something bigger than yourself? Do you feel a sense of belonging where you are or do you struggle with a purpose and direction for your life? Spiritual well-being can also incorporate religion and prayer, which is your personal choice.

All these three areas are equally as important to how you are feeling overall.

Before we begin, I encourage you to think about your own well-being right now. Which aspects are you happy with? Where do you think you would like to make some improvements?

Take some time now to think about all three aspects of your well-being and give each one a score out of ten, in terms of where you feel you currently are today:

1. What is my Mental Well-Being score out of ten?

    •   What is going well?

    _____

    _____

    _____

    _____

- Where would I like to improve?

_____

_____

_____

_____

2. What is my Physical Well-Being score out of ten?

- What is going well?

_____

_____

_____

_____

- Where would I like to improve?

_____

_____

_____

_____

3. What is my Spiritual Well-Being score out of ten?

- What is going well?

_____

_____

_____

_____

- Where would I like to improve?

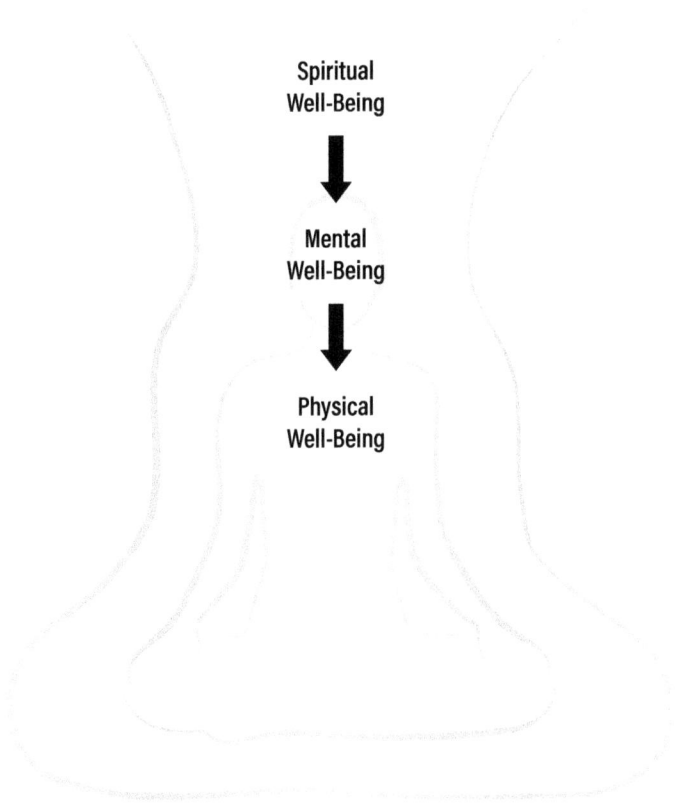

_____

_____

_____

_____

**Spiritual
Well-Being**

⬇

**Mental
Well-Being**

⬇

**Physical
Well-Being**

Multi-Faceted diagram – mind, body, spirit

Completing this exercise will give you a starting point for each aspect. You will also be able to see the area or areas which need(s) more of your focus and attention to help you feel healthy, happy and balanced overall.

Once you start to implement some changes or new activities, it will be useful for you to ask yourself these questions again after 30 days. You can compare your scores and see whether the changes are having a positive impact on your wellness journey.

I would love to hear about your progress. Write to me and let me know how you are getting on. **www.simply-well-being.com**

My Well-Being Journey...

I have not always been interested in the study of well-being. As a child and teenager, the subject was nowhere near my radar! I knew that I should eat healthily and was lucky that this was instilled by my parents.

We always had fruit with our lunch and a balanced dinner with lots of vegetables. Sweets were a treat and only allowed at the weekend. Exercise was an important area in my teenage years; badminton was my sport of choice, mainly because both my parents played for a club and in local leagues. Our family was always in a badminton hall in the evenings or at the weekend. It was a sociable sport and so both myself and my sister learnt to play and joined the same club. It was a social event as much as a sport. We had a lot of friends in this circle and it was very much part of our family life for a long time. I think this is why I enjoyed it so much. Yes, the exercise was good, but the social circle which we enjoyed was probably the best part. Being part of a team and enjoying the company meant that I kept the sport up for many years.

However, mental/psychological well-being was not an area which even featured as a discussion point until I left school. At 18 I wasn't sure I wanted to go to university and so decided to leave school, take a year out and decide what I wanted to do. Moving from the safety, security and routine of school life into the outside world was something which I had not been prepared for at any point during my years at school. Life skills, inner confidence and independent thinking were a far cry from my previous academic syllabus.

With a lack of direction, lack of confidence, lack of self-esteem and feeling like a duck out of water, along came the panic attacks. Anyone who has experienced panic attacks will know that they can be extremely debilitating as well as highly embarrassing. Up until this point, I had been someone who had always been very much in control. I was a straight A student, conscientious, with clear goals and structure and yet suddenly I was feeling out of control, overwhelmed with panic and wanting to run home to the safety of my bedroom. This did little for my confidence at the time. For me it was a culmination of not understanding why the panic attacks had started to happen, not understanding how to make them stop or, indeed, how to handle them. It wasn't long before my mum suggested that I go to see a hypnotherapist. Visiting a hypnotherapist was my first touch point of understanding my mind and the importance of a healthy mind as well as a healthy body.

Over the next few years, alongside work, my interests continued down the holistic path. I completed a number of healing qualifications and loved learning about the spiritual side of humans and how the spirit and the body work together. I qualified as a hypnotherapist myself and I continued my reading and research into the link between mental health and the wellness of our bodies. I've always believed in natural medicines and holistic ways of healing the body where possible. When illness occurs, I believe that this is due to an imbalance somewhere in the body or at a spiritual level. Negative thought patterns can attract physical conditions which aren't wanted as opposed to healthy conditions which are wanted.

I was fascinated by the workings of the mind and to learn and to understand that our mind can be our greatest asset. You may have heard people say that 'mindset' is everything.

I am here to confirm that this is the truth. If you believe you can, then you can. If you believe that you can't, then you can't. Learning how to control your mind so that it works for you and not against you is one of the most important skills to learn in life. It is not easy by any means. I am still learning about this subject 20 years on. It is a journey, it is a process, but it is also extremely rewarding once you comprehend and accept that everything is under your own control.

One of the pinnacle points in my life was investigating alternative birth plans in preparation for when I had my children. On mentioning pregnancy I found that, after the initial congratulations, women are quick to share their horrific birth stories and long lengths of labour as though in competition for who had the worst time of it. I knew that there must be another way and I delivered both my children using HypnoBirthing. HypnoBirthing helps women to deal with any fear or anxiety they may have around birth. It involves education, learning calm breathing techniques, deep relaxation, guided meditation, visualisation and positive affirmations. My births were completely natural with no pain relief, just using the power of the mind and meditation. Therefore, I know and have first-hand experience that alternative techniques do work. We can definitely train our minds to new beliefs. It is our minds which control our bodies and their responses and not the other way around.

Despite my interest and growing knowledge in mental and spiritual well-being, overall holistic well-being was not a concept which I had given much thought to until a couple of years ago.

Every year I was getting older and big birthdays seemed to be creeping up. I was spending a lot of time running around after my children trying to be the perfect mum, the perfect wife, the perfect homemaker and to hold down a job at the same time. There were always a million things on my to do list, the children had numerous after school activities, they needed help with homework, the dog needed walking, shopping still needed doing, and birthdays kept appearing which needed cards and presents. Then there was cooking every evening, endless washing, cleaning, holding down a demanding and stressful job and just generally keeping everything going whilst my husband was travelling. It eventually took its toll. I felt that I had to do everything around the house and for the children, as well as hold down a job. A lot continues to be written on the division of labour in households and I realise that this status quo is hopefully changing. However, I just felt completely exhausted and empty, not just physically but emotionally and spiritually as well. There was nothing medically wrong which doctors could find. There was no reason for my continued exhaustion and after many tests, I was told that I was probably suffering with Chronic Fatigue Syndrome.

(Chronic Fatigue Syndrome is a disorder characterized by extreme fatigue that lasts for at least 6 months and that can't be explained by an underlying medical condition. The fatigue worsens with mental or physical activity but doesn't improve with rest.)

This was a huge wake up call for me. With dependent children who wanted me to be around for a few more years, it was time to take charge and to make some changes. It was time to reduce my stress load, make my daily tasks manageable, look after myself better through food and exercise and to re-connect with my spiritual side again through meditation. Only then did I begin to understand that well-being isn't something which just happens. I had to make it a daily priority in my life and I had to look after each and every aspect of well-being; mind, body and spirit.

It's a process and a journey for all of us. Well-being doesn't just happen overnight. You do have to make the time each day to ensure that you stay on the well-being road.

So, if you are ready, let me help you to get started on this journey.

SECTION ONE

———

Mental Well-Being

Why Mental Health Is So Important

The awareness of mental health has certainly been de-mystified in the past few years. One in four adults experience a mind health issue at some point in their life and, as opposed to being historically very much a taboo subject, it is now becoming a topic which we are encouraged to share and to talk openly about. Over the last few years there have been many media campaigns championing mental health issues, removing the stigma of mental health conditions and encouraging people to seek help and to talk to others.

Whereas historically it might have been viewed as a weakness, and certainly that's how I viewed it in my teenage years, mental health is now a subject which people are coming to feel more comfortable with. Mental health issues can affect anyone at any time; they are not specific to gender or age. Stress, anxiety and the feeling of being totally overwhelmed or out of control can manifest in a number of ways both mentally and physically.

Today our world is consumed by Technology. Everybody is subject to constant messaging, e-mails, texts, WhatsApp's and social media pressure in addition to continuous bombarding of advertising. For some people a mobile phone has become a drug which they seemingly can't live without. A smartphone can be the first thing that is reached for on wakening and the last thing to be checked before going to sleep. Many people experience a constant need to check their phones for fear of missing out on something. But, what could possibly have changed in the last half an hour since they checked it last? Would they really miss anything at all if they just chose to check their social media twice a day? Surely once in the morning and once in the evening would suffice? In reality however, this is easier said than done. This relatively new phone habit is difficult to break and so I will be looking at some activities to help you to unplug from technology in this mental well-being section.

The pace of the working world has hastened in the last 20 years. I'm showing my age when I remember one of my first jobs. I worked in marketing for a paint company in their international department. In order to send a report to every country I would have to stand by the fax machine and fax multiple pages over to our counterparts in various European countries. It was very time consuming. It was also extremely frustrating when the transmission failed and I would have to start all over again! To send the same report today would only take a written e-mail and a quick 'click' to send.

My dad tells the story of how new forms of communication completely changed his working day. He worked in sales and was often on the road driving up and down the country. He originally had a pager which used to ping when someone wanted to speak to him. He would pull into the next service station and make a call on the payphone to solve whatever business issue had arisen. This was his form of mobile communication for many years. As the pace of technology moved on, my dad had one of the very first in-car telephone kits. It was huge, like a brick and I'm sure children today would find it highly amusing. A number of years later he was given a mobile phone. Of course there are many benefits of being contactable 24–7. However, although people believed that mobile technology was moving society forward, my dad said that this advance was coming at a price. The increase in stress within the workplace was also going to ramp up. During his 'pager' days he used his driving time between meetings as thinking time. He could work through issues in his head and come up with solutions. He could relax and de-stress, so that when he arrived at the office he was ready to do his freshest thinking and to participate fully. Fast forward a few years, now armed with his mobile phone and in-car kit, he was constantly available to all customers and employees. He spent the majority of his travelling time on the phone and was also expected to pick up the mobile when he got home too in case of a business emergency. So, what was the result of this change? Increased stress and an overloaded mind. Was more business done? Were more sales made? Probably, but at what price?

Nowadays it may be OK to work at this pace for a period of time, to be on call 24–7 and even to be available during holidays. But can this be sustained for five or six days a week for 45 years? Do we really think that we can function at this highly intense level for so long without there being an issue or two with mental health along the way?

As a mum of two I see the effect of technology on my children. It has been well documented that Millennials are the first generation to be brought up in this new social media world and with it comes many issues and responsibilities. I for one am extremely grateful that Facebook and Instagram were not around when I was in my early 20's. Do I want my friends or employers to be able to see what happened on a girls' holiday to Gran Canaria in 1997? No, I do not! And luckily for me, those stories and photos will remain between myself and my three other girlfriends to remember and laugh about when we get together. My terrible karaoke after a few too many glasses of wine will remain just a memory.

However, the vast majority of the current generation of teens and children are living their entire lives on social media for all to see. This brings with it a whole new level of mental stress. Minimising this stress and teaching children coping strategies and mental health exercises are fundamental to the future mental well-being of our younger generation. There are far too many unrealistic expectations on the youth of today regarding social media, to keep up, to have this app, to post this, to wear that, to look like this, to follow this person, to replicate that etc. I'm feeling quite overwhelmed just writing about it!

For me, it's important to teach strategies which will help people to manage and prioritise their mental health as it is such an important part of our make-up as human beings. Our minds run our bodies and our emotions. So, keeping our minds in check and at peace is a fundamental part of our overall well-being. With the crazy pace of modern life, it is easy to feel out of control as if we are being driven by our environment and outside forces. But the reality is that *we* are in control of our own minds. We can teach them to work for us. We just need to know how. This chapter includes a number of strategies to help you do this.

My Mental Well-Being Journey And Steps Which Help Me

As someone who has suffered with anxiety since my teens, making time to manage my mental well-being is extremely important to me. After my initial hypnotherapy sessions I turned to meditation to help me to control the panic attacks when they arose. I tried a number of different meditation techniques to find which ones I liked and which helped me the most. I found that just meditating for 10–15 minutes most days helped me enormously. Meditation not only helped me to feel calm and in control but, over time, also helped me with my spiritual well-being too. As a busy mum of two, having time out or enjoying my own quiet time is a personal necessity for my mental health. I know I can manage anything which comes my way, as long as I have some quiet meditation time to myself.

Being able to connect to my inner peace (inner peace is

a state of calm despite the presence of outside stress) has helped me through numerous events and situations. The Covid 19 pandemic was one such event. In a matter of days the world literally changed overnight. We were living in Switzerland and during the first few weeks of the pandemic, guidelines of what we could and couldn't do were changing daily. Statistics, hospital deaths, information, do's and don'ts, projections of what was going to happen and predictions of how we would potentially live for an unknown period of time were the only news items and topics of conversation. Everyone was in lockdown and isolating in their homes with no idea of how long this pandemic would last.

It was all extremely unsettling. Personally, I made the mistake of listening to and reading too much media, social media and negative posts. This was very out of character as I hadn't listened to the news for years due to its negative stance. I started to feel anxious and worried for the world we live in. I started worrying and agonising over my children and wondering what effect this pandemic was going to have on their mental health. I forgot my knowledge that there is a huge difference between staying informed and becoming overloaded with negative media.

Once I realised my mistake and identified the reason why I was feeling anxious and out of sorts, I found a daily need to re-connect with my inner peace. I needed to keep myself connected to the stream of Universal Energy which is all around us (Universal Energy is the life force energy around us).

I have continued to find new ways to manage my mental health over the years. Personal development is a passion of mine, so I welcome discovering new ideas and techniques which can potentially help me. Positive affirmations and having an attitude of gratitude have helped me to manifest many new situations, opportunities and desires into my life. I believe

Simply Well-Being

that learning to manage our internal thoughts so that we can manage ourselves is the most powerful skill we can master. It is one which, after all of these years, I am still conquering.

What Does Mental Well-Being Mean To You?

What is your current mental well-being score out of ten? What would you like it to be?

Are you aware of the areas which you would like to improve?

Do you already know some techniques which work for you?

Signs that you need to focus on your mental well-being include, but are not limited to: anxiety, excess worry, panic attacks, mind fog, inability to make decisions, insomnia, confusion, poor memory, feeling sad or down, lack of concentration, an overloaded mind, low energy and tiredness.

There are three main themes which can help you improve your mental well-being and a number of strategies under each theme:

1. **Personal Time** – quiet time, meditation, inner peace.
    Everyone can benefit from some daily, quiet, personal time. Our lives can be so busy and we rush from one thing to the next with a never-ending to-do list. To help limit stress and the feeling of overwhelm, factoring some kind of quiet time into the day helps to calm the mind and subsequently the body. When practised regularly this can help us to feel more relaxed, more peaceful and able to cope with all situations.

2. **Managing Thoughts** – positive self-talk,
   positive affirmations, gratitude, daily wins.
   This is such an important area when discussing mental
   health. Everything is won or lost first and foremost in
   our own mind. If we believe we can, then we can and if
   we believe we can't then we can't, it really is that
   simple. Being aware of and managing our internal
   dialogue so that we become our own biggest
   cheerleader is the key to success.

3. **Connections** – friends and family, calm thinking.
   We are social creatures and are meant to live in
   communities and to be surrounded by others. Finding
   like-minded people with whom we share interests and
   enjoy being with, helps to boost our energy and our
   mental well-being. Spending time doing what we love
   with people we love boosts our overall happiness.

This is not an exhaustive list. As I explained in the introduction, well-being strategies are not mutually exclusive to each other. There are other facets of well-being which can also help with mental well-being such as exercise, sleep, hobbies etc. (see Appendix one for full overview of strategies)

Let's discuss some strategies which can help you improve and strengthen your mental wellness.

1 Quiet Time

Our minds process in excess of 50,000 thoughts a day. That is a lot of thinking! I can't even begin to imagine 50,000 thoughts or what they could possibly consist of. It is therefore no wonder that sometimes we just cannot see what is important and the things that really matter. The benefits of quietening the mind are numerous and help us to not only calm the body, but to think clearly, reduce worry, alleviate stress and, importantly, feel back in control.

Research shows that taking time for silence and calm helps to restore the nervous system, lower blood pressure and decrease the heart rate, reduce muscle tension as well as sustaining energy. Quiet time in summary is a stress eliminator. Do you currently schedule quiet time into your day? Having time just for yourself in every day can be extremely beneficial for your mental health.

No matter how busy your day is, or how many chores and activities you are juggling, everyone can find five minutes in their day to practise some quiet time. Some people say to me that they can finally grab some quiet time when they're driving to work or on their way to pick up the children. This is great and is indeed better than nothing. However, you are still in your conscious mind as you are driving and you need to be paying attention to the road and to the environment around you. So, driving time does not give you the opportunity to completely relax and switch off.

Finding undisturbed quiet time is really what I am talking about here. Even if this is only for five minutes when you get up in the morning, when you're getting ready for bed or when you've arrived somewhere and you can sit in the car by yourself. Deliberate quiet time is where you can completely switch off and let go of all stress and thoughts.

The first rule for your quiet time is to turn off your mobile phone or at least switch it to aeroplane mode. As I have said this needs to be for five whole minutes when you will not be disturbed and you can completely relax. Research has shown that it takes nearly 20 minutes to re-settle and concentrate after hearing a phone ping or vibrate with a new message or notification. We all need periods of time in our day when we switch off all distractions, all emails, messages and all technology. Nothing drastic is going to happen in five minutes.

Now you have 300 seconds of pure, uninterrupted time – what bliss!

TRY THIS EXERCISE...

Read through the exercise first of all and then try it for yourself.

Sit in a comfortable position. Rest your hands in your lap. Place both your feet on the floor. Gently close your eyes and take in a deep breath to a slow count of four ...1...2...3...4 and then breathe out to the count of four ...1...2...3...4.

As you breathe out, relax all of the muscles in your face and let your shoulders and neck relax into the frame of your body. Take in another deep breath again to the count of four and breathe out to the count of four. This time let your chest and stomach relax and sink into your body, so that you are now slouching in your seat. Repeat with a third deep breath, this time letting the relaxation flow down to your legs and feet. Stay in this relaxed position for a few normal breaths and just enjoy the feeling of relaxation. You don't have to be anywhere right now. You don't have to be thinking about anything right now. Just focus on breathing in and breathing out. After a few minutes you can open your eyes.

When you've tried the exercise, how does it make you feel? Do you feel calmer? Do you feel more in control?

This is a very simple exercise which you can do anywhere, in your parked car, on an aeroplane, in a train, just before bed or whilst sitting on your sofa. It's very simple and yet very effective at relaxing your body and quietening your mind. You can set a timer for five minutes if you wish or you can play some relaxing music. You can visualise yourself in your favourite place in nature. Try to find what works best for you. Even practising this five minute period of quiet time can have huge benefits on how you are feeling. For some people five minutes feels like significantly longer when they take the time to finally slow down and just focus on their breathing. Try this simple five minute exercise every day for seven days and see what difference it makes for you.

You can also try this simple exercise multiple times during the day. We can all find many five minute slots throughout our daily routine. To take it further, exaggerate the releasing of muscles and slump down into your chair or wherever you are sitting. You will realise how much tension you were carrying in your neck and shoulders before completing the exercise. Give it a try and see what results you get.

SUGGESTED ACTION

- *schedule five minutes of quiet time each day.*

- *after each session review how you are feeling and whether this exercise has helped you.*

2 Meditation

I have used meditation at various points in my life and I believe it is the key to managing and strengthening our minds. It is possible to condition and train your mind and body to work for you and not against you.

Meditation can help anyone to sustain their health. Whilst technology brings many benefits, the constant need to be online and contactable 24–7 is impacting our mental health in many ways which we are just not even aware of yet. Meditation is the process of calming the mind to a single reference point. It has been proven to calm certain parts of the brain so that the person is focused on the here and now and being in the present moment. The state of your mind matters. Meditation can provide the sense of calm in your otherwise busy and crazy schedules.

There has been a lot of research carried out on the subject of meditation. The effects have been proven to go beyond the period of meditation and can permeate into a person's day, helping them to feel calmer and more in control. Research also suggests that regular meditation practice can make us happier every day.

BENEFITS OF MEDITATION:

- reduces anxiety and stress
- promotes emotional health by providing the opportunity to unplug from technology
- increases focus and lengthens attention spans
- can improve health – by learning to breathe properly your body receives more oxygen and blood pressure can reduce
- can improve the size and strength of your brain
- improves sleep
- can promote feelings of happiness.

As you can see there are numerous benefits to meditating for just a few minutes each day. So, how do you get started?

WHICH TYPE OF MEDITATION SHOULD YOU DO?

There are various types of meditation and my advice is to try a few different forms to see which you like the best. We are all individual and everyone will enjoy certain aspects more than others. Meditation is a personal choice, so be easy about it and have fun finding which one works best for you.

Also, your preferences may change over time depending on what you need during different periods of your life. So, if something is no longer working for you, then feel free to try another type of meditation until you find your new favourite.

Guided Meditation

This, is a good place to start if you've never done meditation before because a guided meditation has someone talking, guiding and leading you on a journey. The journey can take place anywhere. It could take the form of a walk in nature, on the beach, through a rainforest or up a mountain. The guide will ask you to see certain things on your journey as well as challenge you to use your other senses such as touch, smell and taste. All of these senses help you to visualise stronger images in your mind as the meditation progresses.

When you first start meditation, it can be very difficult to quieten the mind. As soon as you stop 'doing' your mind goes into overdrive and numerous thoughts start to flood your mind such as work, activities you think you should be doing, what you need to do next, what you're having for dinner, when you need to pick up the children, or remembering that you need to buy bananas and bread etc. It might well feel as though emptying the mind is just impossible! However, when listening to a guided meditation, the voice and the journey gives your conscious mind something to focus on. It is like you are following a story. Whilst this is happening the chatter in your mind begins to quieten down and your mind and body begin to relax.

Typically, this type of meditation uses background music and helps you to form mental pictures and images which help you to feel relaxed.

You will find that listening to the same guided meditation for a week or two is beneficial in terms of quietening the mind. When the mind hears the same piece of music over and over it begins to associate it with relaxation. When this happens, you will find that your mind and body relax quicker each time you practise this meditation and, as a result, you also go into a deeper state of relaxation. This process is known as conditioning. You are conditioning your mind and body to relax when you hear a specific piece of music.

Your mind quickly creates a neural path associating relaxation in the body with a given trigger, such as music, a voice and breathing patterns. Like any habit, your mind becomes comfortable with the new programme and you can soon see the benefit of daily practise.

When I was practising the HypnoBirthing meditation, I listened to the same meditation most nights for about six months. By the time I came to give birth, just listening to the first few notes of the music from the meditation sent me quickly and easily into a deep state of relaxation. I didn't have to think about it at all. My mind and body just knew that it was relaxation time.

Guided meditation is one of my favourite forms. I have preferred journeys and places in nature where I can take my mind to on any day. When your mind is relaxed, you will find that new thoughts and ideas more easily come to your conscious mind.

Mindfulness Meditation

Mindfulness has gathered popularity over the last few years. As our lives become busier it is commonplace that people are either:

a. living with their minds in the future, thinking about tomorrow, next week and next month.

b. living in the past whilst reflecting on old conversations or what happened yesterday.

Mindfulness focuses on being present in the here and now and enjoying today. Mindfulness Mediation is the process of being fully present with your thoughts right now.

Being mindful means being aware of where you are and what you are doing in the here and now without being distracted by events around you. This can be practised anywhere at any time of the day. Some people prefer to sit in a quiet place, close their eyes and focus on their breathing. But you can choose to be mindful at any point during the day whilst you are walking, driving or doing chores.

TRY THIS EXERCISE...

Stop what you are doing right now and try this.

Bring your attention to the here and now. Notice your five senses. What can you hear, see, smell, taste and touch? How are you feeling in the present moment? What emotion are you feeling? Are you feeling happy or sad? Stop for a few minutes and focus on what is happening around you right here, right now.

This is Mindfulness.

The majority of people have a specific morning routine. Activities are completed in the same order, morning after morning. The brain goes into autopilot. We find that we are not really thinking or concentrating on what we are doing. Our minds are dreaming and are some place other than in the here and now. How many times have you arrived at school or your place of work and yet have no recollection of your journey? This is because your conscious mind was somewhere else either in the past or in the future but definitely not in the active present.

Changing your morning routine or any routine for that matter forces your mind to be fully present and conscious that something different is happening which needs your full attention. Mindfulness meditation is exactly that. It is stopping at points in your day to really focus on the here and now, being fully present in your surroundings and noticing all of your senses.

The power of change is in the here and now. Everything which you are experiencing right now is because of thoughts and beliefs which you had in the past. The Law of Attraction states that what you think about you attract into your life. If you are thinking negative thoughts then you are attracting negativity. Likewise, if you are thinking positive thoughts then you are attracting positivity towards you. The power to change your future and to attract what you want for tomorrow lies with the thoughts which you are thinking right now. You cannot control future or past thoughts, only those which you are thinking this very second.

Mindfulness meditation helps you to identify what you are feeling and thinking in any given moment. If it's not pleasing to you, you have the choice to think a different thought, so that you may be more positive. The moment for change is now.

Mantra Meditation

Mantra Meditation is prominent in many teachings including Hindu and Buddhist traditions. This type of meditation uses a repetitive sound to focus and clear the mind. It can be a word, phrase or sound, whichever appeals to the individual. A popular choice is the word 'Om'.

Om is the highest sacred syllable and, according to Hindu scripture, is the original vibration of the Universe.

The mantra is spoken repeatedly, loudly or quietly. After chanting the mantra for some time, you will be more alert and in tune with your environment. This meditation is good for people who don't like silence and who enjoy repetition. You can listen to music as you are chanting or you can have silence. The choice is yours.

TRY THIS EXERCISE...

Try playing a relaxing soundtrack which is three to five minutes in length. Sit somewhere comfortable, close your eyes and say out loud, "Om". Keep holding the 'mmmmmmmm' sound until the end of your breath. You will find that you automatically find a music note or a resonance as you say the word. Take in a deep breath and then, with every breath out, say the word "Om" again. Repeat this until the end of the track.

How do you feel afterwards? Do you feel calmer? Is your mind clearer? What benefits do you feel?

A good practice to get into is that of writing down how you feel after each meditation. Keep a journal. This will help you to see which meditation type you like best and you will also be able to see your progress over time.

Focused Meditation

Focused Meditation involves choosing one of your five senses and concentrating on it for a period of time. For example, you could use your sight to focus on something tangible like staring at a candle flame. You could close your eyes and use your ears to listen to the sound of the rain on the window. If you're eating a particular food or sucking a sweet, you could close your eyes and focus your entire attention on the taste of whatever it is that you are eating. These are just some examples of a focused meditation. Your full attention should just be on one clear sense for a period of time.

This may sound very simple in theory, but focused meditation can be difficult for beginners. Holding focus on something for any longer than a few minutes can be difficult at first. If your mind wanders, it's important to come back and refocus on the sense which you are studying.

How Can You Get Started With Meditation?

The first step is to decide that you are going to get started and that you are committed to understanding what personal benefits you can gain and enjoy from practising meditation. Set yourself an objective for your meditation. Is your goal to move your mental well-being score from X to Y? Do you want to feel calmer, more in control, happier or more confident?

Whatever your goal, assess how you are feeling before you meditate and re-assess afterwards. Has anything changed?

The second step is to commit to practising. It's best to start your meditation practise in small moments of time, even five or ten minutes to begin with, and build the time up from there. Like most things, meditation takes practise and time to discover what is right for you.

When talking with people about the practise of meditation, some are quick to dismiss it with comments like, "I don't have time to meditate. Do you know how busy I am?" and "I tried it once and it didn't work for me."

Keep a journal and write down how you felt during and after

your practise. Give yourself a score out of ten in terms of where your mental health is before meditating and after meditating. This will help you to identify whether this activity is helping you or not.

Meditation, like most beneficial things, is a skill which needs to be learnt and, like all new skills, takes time and commitment to master. How long did it take you to learn to ride your bike? How many driving lessons and tests did you have before you were allowed to drive on the road by yourself?

All useful life skills take time to learn until they become second nature. In learning anything new, there are certain steps which we all go through. We move from being consciously incompetent (when it is easy to get discouraged and give up) to being unconsciously competent (when the activity is easy and can be done without thinking). Think back to when you were learning to read. You did not wake up one morning able to read perfectly. First of all, you would have learnt your letters, then maybe your phonic sounds and then words. You were probably aware and may have felt a bit impatient at times as you couldn't read the books which you wanted to. Over time you would have read small sentences every day and built up your knowledge of words and meanings. You would have read little and often with your teachers and parents until reading just became second nature. Now you're able to pick up any book without thinking and read it from cover to cover. Your mind goes into auto pilot. Meditation will become like this too given enough time and practise.

Your mind is so used to running at 100 miles per hour and juggling hundreds of thoughts at a time that sitting quietly and trying to calm it can feel impossible in the beginning. But let me reassure you that with practise it will become easier and easier. Over time, you will begin to feel the benefits of this daily quiet time for your mind and you will come to prioritise it more and more. You will begin to look forward to meditating and may even miss it if you don't find time for it during your day.

Like all new activities, it is important to establish a routine if you are to have any chance of creating a habit. It's important to pick a time of day which you will dedicate to your meditation practice. Then you must commit to completing it every day for at least two weeks. This might be first thing in the morning, during your lunch hour, when you get home from work, or maybe last thing at night. However, I would firmly recommend that if you choose to meditate last thing at night, please do not do so in bed as the mind has been conditioned to sleep when you're lying down at the end of the day. Trying to meditate will no doubt just send you to sleep. This is not necessarily a bad thing if sleep is your objective, but you won't feel the full benefit of meditation as you will be sleeping through it. So, my recommendation for nighttime meditation is that you find an alternative, comfortable place such as your sofa or chair. Sit upright, make sure you are warm and comfortable and won't be distracted and then begin whichever meditation type you have chosen.

You may not find meditation easy at first but persevere as it is definitely worth it and the benefits are numerous. I have free meditations on my website to get you started. **www.simply-well-being.com.**

SUGGESTED ACTION

- *if you are a beginner, practise the different types of meditation to find one which works for you. Then meditate once or twice a week for 15 minutes.*

- *if you know meditation then assess what is right for you in terms of time and frequency. Working up to meditating every day for 15 minutes.*

3 Inner Peace

Today more than ever, we need to take time to connect with our inner peace and know that we can do so at any time, in any place and anywhere in the world.

What do I mean by inner peace and Universal Energy?

We are all spiritual beings having a physical experience. We are connected to a much larger universe where there is a constant flow of well-being. We can be connected to it or disconnected, the choice is ours. Meditating and becoming centered enables us to listen to our inner peace. Some call it our inner voice or our inner wisdom or our gut feeling. When we understand that we are part of something bigger than ourselves, that we are part of the universe, that we are spirit in a physical body experiencing the Earth at this time, only then do we begin to realise that we are in control of our lives. By re-connecting to the Universal Energy which is available to everybody, and by replenishing our energy from the universal stream of love and well-being, we can experience a true sense of inner peace and a true sense of what is right for us.

So, how can you connect with your inner peace?

TRY THIS EXERCISE...

Find 10 to 15 minutes, just for yourself. Go outside if you can and reconnect with nature. Sit with your back against a strong tree, or plant yourself cross legged on some grass. Make sure you are in a comfortable position. Close your eyes and take in four deep breaths. Breathe in to the count of four and out to the count of four and repeat. Let your mind begin to relax. Forget everything which is buzzing around your head and just breathe in and out allowing the calm and relaxation to drift down through your body and into the earth, anchoring yourself to Mother Nature. Visualise the relaxation flowing out through your feet and spreading into the ground like roots of a tree. See yourself truly connected now with Mother Nature.

Now, visualise the sky above you being full of positive energy and love. Visualise a stream of this energy flowing down towards you, entering through the top of your head and into your body. Allow this positive energy and love to flow down through your face, your neck, torso, abdomen, legs, knees, ankles and feet. See this positive energy flowing from the sky through your body and down into the ground below.

As you feel the energy drifting down through your body, notice how calm and in control you feel. You can once again feel that, in this moment, all is truly well. Connecting in nature to the Universal Energy like this helps you to connect with your inner voice, your inner wisdom and who you really are. Feel yourself at one with nature. You feel grounded, calm and confident.

Just sit here for a few minutes and enjoy the experience. How are you feeling? What can you hear? What can you see in your mind?

Once you have completed this exercise a couple of times and connected with your inner peace, you can then progress to asking your inner being a question.

When you feel calm and connected to your inner being, you can ask a question, either out loud or in your mind. Ask any question which you have been pondering over or which you would like an answer to and trust the first answer, thought or idea which comes into your head. Don't overthink or analyse what comes to mind. Just remember the first thing which comes into your mind when you ask that question. This answer has come from your inner wisdom. Some say this comes from your spirit guides, your angels, your god or the universe. Whatever you believe in, this is your inner wisdom communicating with you.

When we quieten our conscious minds and open our subconscious minds we find answers and solutions to many, many questions. During the everyday it's our conscious minds which run our lives by analysing, over thinking and remembering what has gone before. Sometimes we can struggle to come up with new ideas and solutions. By taking time out to calm and relax our minds we can connect with our inner peace and wisdom to feel and hear what is right for us in this very moment. If the answer or thought feels good then it is the right decision or the right direction for you to take.

Remember that you are in control of your thoughts and you are also in control of your immediate environment. This exercise in nature is a great place to start and to re-connect with who you really are.

SUGGESTED ACTION

- *Connect with nature twice a week.*
- *Connect with nature daily.*

4 Positive Self-Talk

Have you ever sat and listened to the ongoing conversations and thoughts in your head? Throughout the day we all have a constant dialogue going on in our head. This may include thoughts about what is happening around us, what people are saying, what we can see, what we think on key subjects, what we're having for dinner, where we shall go on holiday next year, or whether we remembered to send our Auntie a birthday card etc. Our minds experience in excess of 50,000 thoughts in a day!

All of these inner thoughts and conversations are either positive or negative. As adult human beings our minds seem to have become conditioned to more readily believe or tune into negativity rather than positivity. The reason for this is that negative events have a greater impact on our minds than positive ones. Psychologists refer to this as the negative bias. This can be especially true when we hear people's opinions of us or when people comment on what choices we have made or whether they agree with what we are doing. It can be easier to believe and fixate on a negative comment as opposed to trusting, believing and building on positive comments.

Take a few minutes to reflect on this and decide whether this is true for you. When someone pays you a compliment do you say, "Thank you" and feel good for the rest of the day? Or do you quickly turn it into something negative?

If someone says, "Oh you've had your hair cut. It looks nice." Is your reply, "Thanks but my hairdresser cut it too short. It wasn't really what I asked for."?

Or perhaps a friend observes, "That dress looks great on you." and your reply is, "Thanks but I'm not sure it's really my colour."

Or maybe a colleague congratulates you by saying, "You did a great job delivering that presentation!" but you reply, "Thanks but I forgot to say so many key points and I messed up the summary."

Is this what you do? As opposed to accepting the compliment graciously, do you turn it into a negative comment because it makes you feel more comfortable?

A person's mindset is a set of beliefs that shapes how they see themselves and how they make sense of the world around them. Everyone sees life through their own unique lens. Research shows that mindset plays a significant role in determining our life outcome. And the good news is that mindsets are changeable and we can learn to re-program them so that we can attract the life we want.

When faced with a new task or something you haven't done before do you find yourself saying, "Great I can do this. Let's give it a go!" or are you in the camp of, "I'm too old. I don't like trying new things. I won't be able to do this."?

Our internal dialogue is influenced by a lot of external factors, including other people's opinions. This will constrain us unless we decide to take control of this banter in our heads and ensure that our minds and thoughts are working for us and not against us.

You must become your own biggest cheerleader in life because, no one else is going to play this role for you. You may have parents who are always cheering you on or good friends who are encouraging and supporting you but, ultimately, it's what you think and say to yourself which is so vitally important to your mental well-being. It is your own minute-by-minute self-talk which is either building you up or taking you down. Think about this for a minute. Why would you intentionally talk yourself down? Why would you intentionally say to yourself that you can't do something? Why would you intentionally criticise yourself?

And yet many of us do this all the time as it feels more comfortable to us. Perhaps it feels easier to be negative and expect the worst as then we can't be disappointed if we don't get the outcome which we really want.

First and foremost and without exception, the challenge, dream or goal is won or lost in your head. In order to achieve whatever you set out to accomplish, you have to believe that you can. It all comes down to mindset.

I don't believe that we are intentionally negative or that we set out with the objective of sabotaging our own hopes and aspirations. I just think that we aren't aware that a lot of our self-talk and inner dialogue is negative. Many of us just aren't aware of this negativity bias which humans lean towards.

Take a moment to reflect. Is your self-talk positive or negative?

When something doesn't go right in your day, do you think, "That was all my fault. I deserved that?" or do you think, "What can I learn from this? How did this happen? Why did this happen?"

When you go for a new job or try something new and it doesn't work out, do you think, "I'm not good enough!" or, "People never take me seriously!" or, "I'm just not good at this!"? Or do you think, "Something better is just around the corner for me."?

Take some time to stop and evaluate your daily thoughts

and identify whether the majority of your thoughts about yourself are positive or negative? Are you cheering yourself on or are you feeding your self-doubt?

With tens of thousands of thoughts crossing your mind each day, you can't possibly control them all. However, you can control, or at least make the conscious effort to control, the overall balance of your thoughts. You can choose to be a cup half-full type of person and not a cup half-empty. You just have to be aware in the moment of what you are thinking and be willing to make a conscious change.

So, how can you change your self-talk?

The first step you need to take is to be aware of what you are saying and how you are talking to yourself. Negative self-talk falls into three main categories:

1. **Self-Sabotage** – you blame yourself for everything which happens to you.

2. **Amplifying** – during a situation you think about all of the negative aspects and ignore any positives which there might be.

3. **Dramatising** – before a situation or event happens you are expecting the worst.

Once you identify the negative self-talk, the second step is to turn that thought into a positive one.

Self Sabotage

I knew this would happen to me...	...What can I learn from this?
I am just not good enough...	...I am good enough.
I knew I couldn't do this...	...I do not know how to do this yet.
What was I thinking?...	...I am proud that I gave it a go.
I'm a failure...	...What can I do differently next time?

Amplifying

This is going to end in disaster...	...What could be a positive outcome?
I always have issues when I travel...	...What would my perfect journey look like?
I missed my train and now my whole day is ruined...	...How can I rearrange this to my advantage?

Dramatising

I'm going to fail...	...I will do my best and ask for help with...
Everyone else is so much better...	...I am doing my best, I am unique.
I am sure no one will turn up to the party...	...The party will be fun regardless.

Turning negative thoughts into positive ones takes time and does not happen overnight. The first step is being aware that the negative thoughts are happening. When you are aware of what you are thinking you can pause, reflect and then consciously turn that thought into a positive one which you can repeat over and over.

TRY THIS EXERCISE...

Start by taking one day. Stop at various intervals to assess what you are thinking and whether it is positive or negative. You could set an alarm for every hour, or stick Post-It notes in various rooms so that when you see the reminder, you stop and analyse your thoughts.

Find a system that works for you, but make sure you stop and assess your thoughts at least ten times during the day. You might be surprised by your thoughts. Jot them down. Identify if you could adopt a more positive thought instead. This does take effort, but it is a very interesting exercise to do.

Positive self-talk can have a huge impact on your daily well-being and this leads nicely to my next section about Positive Affirmations. These two topics go hand-in-hand. It can help immensely if you have some positive affirmations to hand when you realise that negative self-talk is happening.

SUGGESTED ACTION

- *Stop yourself ten times a day to assess whether your thoughts are positive or negative.*

- *Consciously turn your thoughts into positive ones.*

Conscious Mind

Subconscious Mind

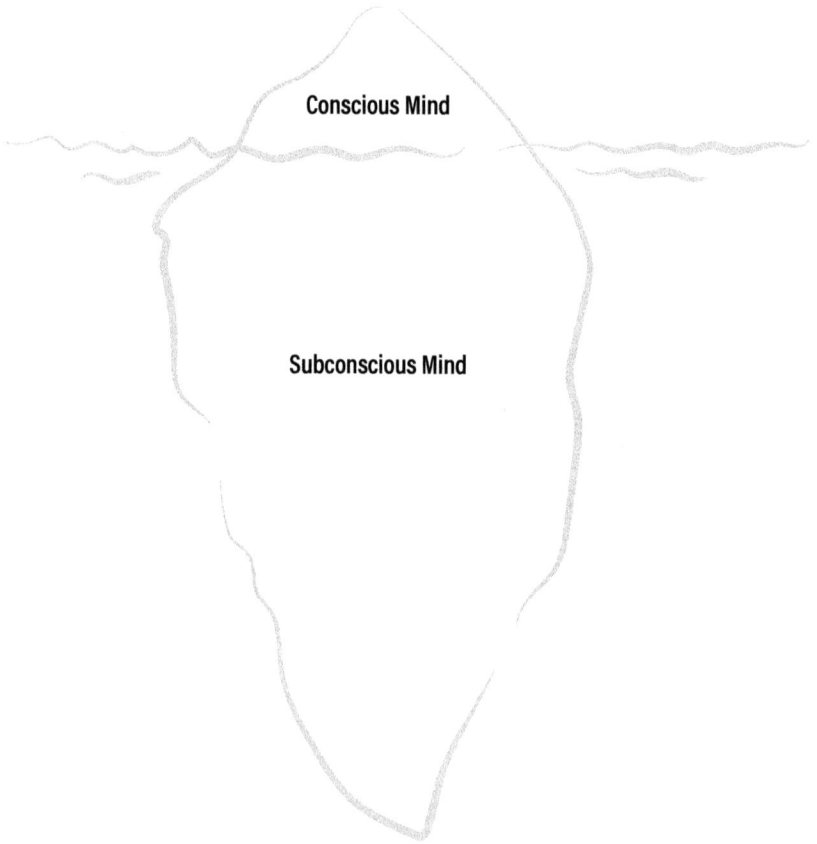

Iceberg diagram

5 Positive Affirmations

90% of our brain activity is beyond our conscious awareness. Sit and ponder on this for a moment. Our minds really are as vast as the sky and hold every experience and memory from the day you were born right up to what has happened to you today. However, the majority of these millions of experiences and memories are not readily available to us as conscious thoughts on a day-to-day basis. So, what does this mean for our daily experience?

Having 90% of your brain activity as subconscious thought means that your daily conscious experiences are largely affected by your subconscious beliefs, attitudes, and behaviours. (see Iceberg Diagram) These subconscious beliefs, attitudes and behaviours may be working for you or they may be working against you. For example, you might have picked up some limiting beliefs during your childhood which are no longer serving you as an adult. You may have been repeatedly told something over and over as a child or teenager which is no longer true for you as an adult. Often if there is an area in your life which is blocked or not working for you on some level, when you dig into the reasons underlying the problem or issue, nine times out of ten it is linked to beliefs which your subconscious mind is holding onto and, which are preventing you from moving forward or hindering you from making the changes which you want in your life.

Everyone has different beliefs and motivations, but a lot of beliefs which are stored in our subconscious are a result of what we have seen, been told or been led to believe as we were growing up. These beliefs may not be serving us today. So, let's analyse what a belief actually is.

A belief is a thought which exists and which you have accepted to be true.

Some beliefs will be serving you well and keeping you safe, but some will no longer be helpful for you and it's important to understand which ones you want to continue believing and which ones you don't.

For example, I believe that I shouldn't put my hand in a fire as I will get burnt. This is probably a very good belief to keep in my subconscious. I don't need to consciously think about this. When I'm near a fire I know to instinctively keep my distance and not to get too close. This belief is keeping me safe from harm.

Let's look at another example. I believe that electricity and water do not mix. I therefore know subconsciously not to let electrical devices anywhere near a sink full of water, a bath or any other volume of water otherwise I will be electrocuted. This is also a belief which I am happy to keep as it protects me from potential harm.

However, another example could be that I believe that money doesn't grow on trees and that I will have to work hard for a living. Some people will accept this belief. They may have resigned themselves to the fact that they will have to work hard their entire lives. But what if you wanted to change this belief? What if this is the belief which is holding you back in your life? What if this is the belief which is causing you to have financial worries? Can you change this belief to something else?

The simple answer is, yes, you can.

You can change this belief and re-wire your mind. You can

tell your conscious and subconscious minds a different story and choose to believe a different thought. A belief is just a thought which you have accepted to be true so, in order to change the belief, you need to change your thought. You must believe that this new thought is true for you and repeat it over and over until it becomes your new truth and your new belief.

Look around and identify people who don't have to work hard for a living and who have money flowing to them from multiple directions. Now you can see evidence that there are people who are not limited by a belief that they have to work hard for a living. It is clearly not a belief for everyone. It is not a Universal Law and therefore you don't have to be limited by this belief either. You have a choice.

In order to change your belief, you have to change your conscious thoughts, and you have to repeat the new thoughts over and over again. You also have to believe that this new thought is true for you. Examples of new thoughts which you could choose are:

- Money flows easily to me.

- I love my work and it is a joy to me.

- My work is fun, easy and fulfilling.

- I earn a full-time salary working part-time.

These new positive statements are also known as positive affirmations and they help to shift unwanted subconscious thoughts and experiences into positive ones. By writing these positive statements down and repeating them over and over again, you can change your thoughts. These new thoughts become new beliefs and this can lead to real positive change in your life.

Positive affirmations are very easy to construct once you understand the rules and know what they should and shouldn't include. There are six considerations which I will share with you so that your affirmations are as effective as possible:

1. **Positive affirmations should be positive – avoid negatives.** The human mind struggles to comprehend the negative. For example, if I said to you, "Don't think of a tiger," what have you just thought of? A tiger! New research suggests that how the brain interprets the statement does depend on where the negative is in the sentence. However, as this is a complex area, it is best that positive affirmations are purely positive. Always avoid negatives or double negatives. If you say, "I don't want to be sick," the brain can only understand the "want to be sick" element of that statement. It does not understand "don't". So, you need to state what you do want and not what you don't want. Keep your affirmations positive, e.g. I am healthy. My body is healthy and well. I am full of energy etc.

2. **Always use the present tense when saying positive affirmations**. The mind is a very powerful tool and it seeks to manifest what it believes. By speaking in the present tense you are stating that the affirmation already exists and that it is already true for you. This helps the mind to manifest the affirmation in a shorter time period. If we state something in the future, the mind has no concept of time and can therefore get confused. By saying, "I will find someone who loves me just as I am," can mean that you want this to manifest at any time in your life, even when you are 99 years old! By stating your desire in the present tense however and saying, "I am loved by someone who loves me just as I am," you are stating that you are loved right now and

Simply Well-Being

that your desire is true now and not at some point in the future. This helps the mind to manifest your desire in the here and now.

3. **Create positive affirmations that focus on the solution and not the problem.** You want to give your conscious and subconscious minds a clear picture of what you do want and therefore you need to ensure that your affirmations are focused on the solution and the outcome which you are wanting and expecting. If you state, "I don't want to fail my driving test," your brain hears "fail my driving test." The statement needs to be rewritten to focus on the desired outcome, "I pass my driving test with ease." Can you see the difference?

4. **Write positive affirmations that are specific, simple, and direct.** Writing an essay or paragraph is not going to be easy to remember and will confuse the brain as to what it is that you actually want! So, keep your affirmations short, punchy and to the point. They should be easy to remember so that you can recite them over and over again. The brain understands simple, clear instructions. Once you have written your affirmations, test them by going through each of these first four guidelines to make sure they are as effective as you need them to be.

5. **Fill your positive affirmations with passion and add visualisations.** Say your affirmations outloud and with conviction. Even if they are not yet true for you, believe that they are. Believe that they have already manifested in your life. When you say them out loud, visualise them in your mind as already happening. Visualisation is a

powerful tool used by many. Athletes visualise their race or event before the start. They see themselves winning, running the fastest and jumping the highest or longest. When they do this, their chances of success increase dramatically. So, visualising having or being what you're saying helps the mind to manifest the reality in a shorter timeframe.

Sometimes we need to change our beliefs in small steps. This is especially so if the new belief which we would like is very different from our current reality. For example, someone who is overweight may have the goal of being a size 12.

Scenario one – the person is currently a size 14. Their new affirmation may be, "I am a perfect size 12." "Size 12 clothes fit me with ease." If this person visualises themself as a size 12 and believes that this is possible, then the affirmations are good.

Scenario two – the person is currently a size 18. Their new affirmations of "I am a perfect size 12" and "Size 12 clothes fit me with ease," are very different from this person's current reality. In this instance, smaller, more general affirmations would be better, such as, "My body enjoys the healthy food which I eat", "I'm really excited about buying new size 16 clothes" and "I am happy and healthy and approve of my body". Over time as this person gets closer to their goal of being a size 12, they can change their affirmations.

For positive affirmations to work, you must feel that they are right for you and you must feel that they are true for you. If not, then you need to re-write them to something which is closer to where you are now. Don't try and jump too far in one go.

Useful phrases to help you with this are:

"Wouldn't it be nice if..."
"I'm really excited about..."

6. **Start your positive affirmation practice and keep consistent.** Finding a time each day to say and recite your affirmations is key. To see results, you need to make positive affirmations a habit and therefore, you need to find a time of day which works for you and commit to it without fail. My favourite times are first thing in the morning before I get out of bed or whilst I'm brushing my teeth. It's also powerful to say your affirmations just as you're drifting off to sleep, so that the last conscious memory are your positive affirmations. If you've never said affirmations before then you may feel a bit reluctant to begin with. My advice is to set yourself a goal of saying two to three affirmations every day for 30 days. Review after 30 days. How are you feeling? Are you enjoying the affirmations? Are you feeling more positive? Has anything tangibly changed yet as a result? Are the affirmations still right for you? Are there any which you would like to add to your list? Review the six considerations above to ensure that your affirmations are constructed correctly.

Positive affirmations can be used for any aspect of your life including, relationships, health, fitness, work, school, confidence, balance, money etc. To get you started, choose one or two subjects where you would like to make a change. What are your current thoughts on the subject? What would you like to be true instead? From this information, create a positive statement. It really is quite simple once you have done this a couple of times. You can add to your affirmations, change them and include more subjects as you get going. For me, the best outcomes I have experienced is when I have had two to three key affirmations. I have learnt them off by heart and therefore can chant them over and over in my head during the day as I'm going about my daily business. After 30 days I have experienced a shift in beliefs, an increase in energy for a specific subject, as well as manifesting events and solutions in my life.

TRY THIS EXERCISE...

Stop right now and find yourself a mirror. Look yourself in the eye and repeat this statement out loud three times : I am wonderful. I am unique. I am enough.

How did that make you feel? Did you believe yourself as you were speaking? Did that make you feel happy or uncomfortable?

All three of these statements are true about you, but if you felt uncomfortable you may just not believe them right now. If that is the case, then just choose the one which you do believe about yourself. Go back to the mirror and just repeat this one statement. Is that better?

To get you started, here are some of my favourite positive affirmations, but please make them specific for you.

All is well.

I am happy and healthy.

Everything is working out for me.

I make a difference where I can.

I work with people who love and respect me.

Every day I strive to be better.

I believe in, trust and have confidence in myself.

I eat well, exercise regularly and get plenty of rest to enjoy good health.

I can accomplish anything I set my mind to.

I am good at my job and love helping people.

Money flows effortlessly into my life.

I'm worthy of abundance.

I am kind and do good every day.

I am proud of myself for...

I believe in myself and my ability to succeed.

I am doing a great job.

I am enough.

Write down your positive statements, save them on a Post-It note or on your smartphone so that you have them to hand throughout the day. Just repeating your affirmations two or three times a day can have a really positive effect over time.

SUGGESTED ACTION

- *Write three Positive Affirmations and repeat them three times a day for 30 days.*

- *Record how you feel day one, day seven and also day 30.*

6 Attitude of Gratitude

The Law of Attraction is a universal principle which states that you will attract into your life that which you focus on. The law is a given, it cannot be altered or changed and it works every single time without question. A law is something that works whether you believe in it or not and it also exists before you know about it. Gravity for example, was in existence before Newton discovered it and named it the law of universal gravitation, it does not rely on your beliefs for it to function.

Quantum Physics tells us that everything vibrates, everything is energy and our entire universe is pure energy. For those questioning this concept, let's look at the science. Take any everyday object and put it under a microscope. In most cases this will need to be an extremely powerful microscope. Scientists have proven that at the core of any solid, liquid or gas you will find molecules, atoms, protons, neutrons and electrons. Scientists have also proven that all of these are vibrating energy at their core. There are a multitude of different vibrations or waves of energy from extremely slow to ultra-fast but nonetheless, everything which is in our environment, from plants, flowers, buildings and cars to ourselves as human beings, is all just vibrating energy at its core.

Our thoughts and feelings also have their own energy or

vibration. We cannot necessarily see the energy, but we can feel it if we sit and tune into our thoughts and feelings.

Let's look at some examples which demonstrate the law of attraction.

- Typically a person who is miserable and complains a lot, will attract friends or followers who have a bad attitude.

- Typically a person who is happy and positive will attract other enthusiastic, kind friends into their life.

This can be summarised by the phrase, 'birds of a feather flock together.' Humans like to be around other people who are 'like them.'

Whatever vibration you emanate out to the world, you will receive back in the form of experiences or objects those which are on the same vibrational platform as that which you are projecting.

'What you think about, you bring about.'

'What you put out into the universe you receive.'

All thoughts which you are thinking have their own vibration. As discussed previously, you can either be thinking positive thoughts or negative thoughts. To illustrate the law of attraction in simple terms, positive thoughts will attract more positive ones and conversely negative thoughts will attract more negative ones.

Once you have an understanding of the law of attraction, you can understand the benefits of having an attitude of gratitude. When you express gratitude openly and verbally, you are basically saying to the universe, "Thank you so much for XYZ. I'd like some more of this please." Taking time to appreciate everything which you are grateful for focuses your mind and thoughts on a positive trajectory. When you continue having an attitude of gratitude, this in turn attracts more things in your life to be grateful for.

The evening is a great time to reflect on your day and to remember all of those things which you are grateful for. These appreciations can be endless because, regardless of your situation, you can always find something to be grateful for. Some topics to get you started could include events, experiences, family, friends, colleagues, food and water, where you live, possessions, time, your environment, the weather, money and health. Don't be afraid to drill down and go into specifics for each area.

Having a Gratitude Journal which you write in each evening may help you to keep this daily habit on track. Without a place to write your appreciations and thoughts, it's easy to just forget to do this gratitude exercise at the end of the day. For example, I have a book on my bedside table which reminds me to do this every evening.

As well as writing three to five things which I am grateful for every day, I then think of the one thing which I'm most grateful for in each day. This helps me to focus on one specific thing which has happened that day and which I am extremely appreciative of. It's important to think of new things to be thankful for each day as opposed to writing the same things day in and day out.

You might find it helpful to focus on a specific topic each week or each day of the week. For example, one week I focused on health and every day I wrote down specifics such as how grateful I was for my eyesight to see objects and colour, for my hands and fingers which help me in everything I do throughout the day and for my feet and toes which provide me with balance and help to get me from A to B every day but which are normally overlooked.

Challenge yourself to get creative. Once you start thinking about all of the things, great and small, which you are grateful for, you will be absolutely amazed by the list which you come up with. Try each day to think of three to five different things which you are thankful for. Hopefully this will not be too difficult.

So, why do I recommend that you do this activity at nighttime?

Our minds wake up each morning on the same vibration as when we went to sleep. I remember my mum advising me never to go to bed angry and never to go to bed after a fight. You might think that you will wake in the morning feeling better, but, in reality, when you wake and come back into your conscious mind, your first waking thought is often the last one from the night before. Therefore, if you have gone to bed feeling angry and still going over the points of an argument in your head, the anger all comes flooding back as soon as you awake. This means that now you are starting the day on a negative vibration.

So, by recalling what you are grateful for before falling asleep you project positive vibrations which will carry through to the morning. This means that you awake on a positive vibration which, in my opinion, is the best way to start any day.

Of course, it's not just in the evening when having an attitude of gratitude works. When you're mindful of being grateful during the day, the process is just as powerful. Spending a few minutes before you get out of bed each morning is also a great time to practice gratitude. Think of what you were thankful for the previous day, then think about all of the great things which you want to happen during this day and all of the things which you will be giving thanks for before you go to bed that evening. If you can't think of specifics for your day then just think some generic positive thoughts to start your day, such as, "Today is

Simply Well-Being

going to be a great day!", "Today, everything will work out well for me", or, "All is well." These are all great phrases to say out loud to start your day on a positive vibration.

TRY THIS EXERCISE...

Stop right now and write down three things which you are grateful for today.

How did you find that? Did you easily think of three things or did it take you a while?

When you are aware of being grateful and expressing thanks, there will be many times during the day when a situation will present itself to you. For example, when traffic lights turn green for you, when your meeting goes well, when you get a good mark on your assignment, when someone pays you a compliment, when a friend calls you from out of the blue or when you sit down to eat a meal. The occasions are endless. Once you get into the habit of having an attitude of gratitude, it is fun and you will also notice more and more things to be grateful for. The flow of well-being is never-ending.

On some days you may be struggling to be positive. We all have those days when things just aren't going as well as we'd like. We feel tired, fed up and irritable. Speaking from my personal experience, it can seem hard to pivot and change our vibration to a more positive one, but it is definitely a skill worth mastering. During challenging times if you can find just one thing to be grateful for and, if you express your gratitude for this one thing out loud, your vibration will begin to shift in a positive direction. If you can hold a positive thought for long enough, then another one will appear and then another. So, next time you are feeling a bit fed up or less than positive, as opposed to spiraling down further with more negative thoughts, stop.

Acknowledge what you are feeling and try your hardest to find something to be thankful for. However small it may be, hold that gratitude thought and wait for the next one to appear. Congratulate yourself on finding a new positive focus.

I've started the practice of gratitude with my children as I believe that they are never too young to start. Every night at bedtime I ask them what has gone well today and what they are grateful for. In the beginning, they both found this a strange and difficult exercise to do. But once they started, it became easier and they now have no problem at all thinking of at least one thing which they are thankful for each day. For younger children, why not paint a large tree together and put it on their wall? Each night they can write on it something they are grateful for that day. Over time they will have a tree bursting with positivity.

The gratitude process literally takes only a few minutes out of your day but the results can be huge. Try it and see. Let me know how you get on. Purchase a nice notebook to keep beside your bed. It will act as a reminder before you turn the light out that you need to write down your list of appreciations. Commit to doing this for 30 days and see how you feel. Having an attitude of gratitude is the best daily habit you can create for your mental well-being.

Here are some examples of daily gratitude:

- I am grateful for my health and feeling energised today.

- I am grateful for living in this beautiful part of the world.

- I am grateful for my house which is providing such a happy home.

- I am grateful for the healthy food which I ate today.

- I am grateful for the time I spent with my children today, it was great when we...

- I am grateful for clean running water ... etc.

SUGGESTED ACTION

- *Buy yourself a gratitude journal.*
- *Write down what you are grateful for each day.*

7 Daily Wins

One of the downsides of the crazy 100mph lives which a lot of people seem to lead these days is that people are too busy to sit and reflect on how well they are doing. We can be so focused on our huge 'to do' list (which, by the way, is like your Facebook news feed: never-ending) that we can sometimes feel like we aren't getting anywhere.

Do you ever get to the end of the week and wonder where it went? Do you ever wonder what you have actually achieved when Friday rolls around again? Do you have goals which you don't feel like you're getting any closer to?

It can feel overwhelming when you have so much to do all of the time, when you feel so busy that you don't have time to stop and breathe. You feel like you are on a continuous treadmill which you can't get off and you can start to feel discouraged. The reality is that you are achieving more in a day than you realise. You will feel more relaxed and contented by slowing down and taking note of all the individual activities which you do accomplish each day, as well as giving yourself credit for managing your mental and physical health.

It is also true that we have a tendency to focus on what's not going well rather than what is going well. For example, you could have had a perfectly good day but maybe made one small mistake. You are likely to be re-living the mistake over and over again as opposed to congratulating yourself on the hundreds of things which went well. The human mind is quick to punish and very slow to celebrate good performance.

Reflecting on your wins helps you to feel good, to feel positive and to feel motivated. When you know that you are making progress it feels great and is highly motivating. Your confidence is boosted and this helps you to keep pushing forward.

People around you are too busy with their own lives to notice your achievements. You need to become your own biggest cheerleader. Only you can record your daily victories.

Having worked in Corporate Marketing for over 20 years, I used to work crazy hours. I could juggle 20 projects, deliver a five-star market-wide launch, speak at a conference, co-ordinate multiple agencies and manage my team. However, I felt constantly stressed. My mind rarely switched off. I was worried about whether I was doing a good enough job and I was continuously exhausted. People rarely complimented me on my performance and I hardly ever stopped to take note of my achievements. Looking back, my self-esteem should have been high, but it wasn't. I just wasn't cheering myself on. I wasn't celebrating my wins and successes.

You need to start appreciating yourself for everything which you are achieving daily both mentally and physically. You need to acknowledge what makes you great.

One way to do this is to record your daily wins at the end of the day. This is not just about recording specific actions which you have completed during the day but also about how you felt, what your mental state was throughout the day and how you felt physically. You win and flourish in life when all areas of yourself are in balance. It is not just about what you do but also how you feel whilst doing the actions. So, give yourself a score out of 10 or 100 for how you felt physically as well as mentally during the day. Keeping calm when things have

Simply Well-Being

not gone to plan at work or at home is a huge win which you should acknowledge and be proud of. Feeling positive when not everything is happening as fast as you would like is also a huge win and should be celebrated.

I use my Gratitude Journal for this exercise. One end of the book is for me to record gratitude and the other end for recording my daily wins. At the end of each day, I will record small wins such as completing the shopping, ordering birthday presents or walking the dog for an hour. I will also write my business wins such as winning a new customer, reaching out to 20 people or spending two hours working on my book. And finally, I will also write how I felt during the day. For example, I felt energized, I felt content, I felt a bit bored, I felt happy, I felt calm etc.

TRY THIS EXERCISE...

Stop right now and write down at least two wins which you have achieved today so far. They can be anything, big or small.

Acknowledging small daily wins helps our minds to be more motivated and can also lead to higher self-esteem. It's a great feeling to read through your daily wins and surprising too, when you realise just how much you have accomplished both in terms of actions and also in terms of your mindset and emotions.

So, I would encourage you to add this to your daily routine. After you have written your daily gratitude list, turn to the back of your book and start a daily win section. Not only will this be a lovely, positive list, but hopefully you will also be able to see improvements in your physical and mental well-being as you continue over time.

Examples:

- got the children up, fed and to school on time
- did the shopping
- completed the conference presentation
- went for a walk at lunchtime
- drank 1.5 litres of water
- had a lovely catch up with a dear friend
- did a workout / went to the gym
- felt energized all day
- kept calm even when...

SUGGESTED ACTION

- *write down your daily wins at the end of each day for 30 days. Reflect how you feel at the end of the 30 days.*

8 Friends And Family

For any of you from the UK, you may remember the British Telecom adverts in the nineties. Their strapline was, "It's good to talk." Simple but so true, even today.

We are a social species. Human beings have always lived in communities and formed social groups. We are built to seek social companionship; this is how we live and this is how our species has survived. Maslow's Hierarchy of Needs states that after our physiological needs (air, food, water, shelter, clothing) and safety needs (personal security, health) are met, the next most important human need is love and belonging and a sense of connection.

There is a lot of research in this area which concludes that being around other people makes us healthier. Physiologically, the absence of a social support system is a source of stress for our bodies. Studies have also shown that when people feel lonely, they have higher levels of the stress hormone cortisol. The human brain expects social relationships. Think back to species survival and safety in numbers. Isn't it true that just having another person with you who you trust and who you feel safe around can help to make the world look like a less-challenging place?

Therefore, it is important for positive mental well-being to ensure that you are spending time in the company of others. Since having children, I have been lucky enough to have had a couple of roles which were home-based. These roles gave me great flexibility in terms of being able to pick my children up from school most days. However, after a while I noticed that my daily mood had changed and I realised that, although I was speaking to people on the phone every day, not being surrounded by people and not having the company of others was making me feel sad and lethargic. That was when I knew that it was time to get back to an office environment.

The Covid pandemic has definitely changed the way in which people work. A lot of companies no longer expect employees to be in the office five days a week. Home-based working has become the norm for a lot of people and does offer many benefits, especially for working parents. However, as a wellness coach my preference for people is definitely a hybrid working model. It's important to build face-to-face relationships and it's important to interact face-to-face as well.

I'm often asked whether this is true for introverts as well as extroverts and the answer is, yes. Everyone needs social interaction in their lives. Extroverts may well need more interaction with a larger volume of people, as this is where they get their energy from, but introverts also need social time with others, although they may only need one or two people.

So, when you are assessing your daily mental well-being, keep social interactions high on your agenda. Some days all the therapy you need is to speak to a friend. "A problem shared is a problem halved." "Laughter is the best medicine." Both of these sayings demonstrate the power of companionship and being with people.

TRY THIS EXERCISE...

Think of the best times in your life? Were you alone or who were you with? What made those times so amazing?

I'm going to guess that you remembered events which you have shared with at least one other person.

What's the one thing you want to do when you receive some good news? When you passed your exams, got offered a job, got engaged or found out you were going to be a parent? What did you do? I will hazard a guess that your first instinct was to phone someone such as your mum, your dad, your best friend or your partner. You wanted to share the good news with your nearest and dearest and the people who are most important in your life. We are social beings and meant to share our lives with other people.

Hobbies and interests are an essential part of who you are. Feeling connected with like-minded people who share your interests makes you happy. Doing something you enjoy every day will always lift your mood and improve your mental well-being. What hobbies do you have? What do you enjoy doing? What do you do for yourself every day?

Maybe you are part of your local football or netball team. Playing a team sport will help you both physically and mentally. Maybe you love reading and are part of a book club or you love being onstage and so have joined your local amateur society group. Maybe you love walking with a friend or playing chess. Whatever you love to do in your spare time, being around other people or just one other person will help to satisfy your need for human connection and bonding.

So, to boost your mental well-being, make sure that you are meeting people regularly. Schedule that coffee or drink with a friend. Pick up the phone and speak to your mum, dad, sister or brother. Keep connecting with people. Be selfish. Prioritise your hobbies and your social life. Keep talking and keep laughing. Your mental well-being will be happier for it.

SUGGESTED ACTION

- *Look at your weekly schedule and decide if you have enough friends and family time allocated. If not, then change your plan. Add in more phone calls, more face-to-face get-togethers.*

- *If your mental well-being score was low and you decided to reach out to friends or family, how did you feel afterwards? What was your mental well-being score after the interaction?*

Hopefully, you can see a positive correlation as chatter does matter!

9 Calm Thinking

Have you ever had one of those days when you have so much buzzing around inside of your head that you just can't see the wood for the trees? When you feel completely overwhelmed and don't know where to start?

Have you ever struggled to make a decision on an important matter? You keep arguing all sides in your head but you just can't decide what is right for you.

These and other scenarios can happen when you are suffering from mental stress. You can feel overwhelmed, worried, anxious and not too sure which way to turn.

In these situations, a lot of people may turn to others for advice. How many times have you asked your mum or dad for their opinion? Or, how many times have you phoned a friend to ask what they would do in your situation?

Sometimes, if you are lucky, the person you have asked may well give you some good advice which makes sense to you. But have you ever had someone advise you what to do only for it not to sit well with you? Only for you to then think, "This person doesn't know me at all," or, "That is definitely not what I'm going to do"?

Friends, family and advisors may try their best to help you, to give advice as to what they would do in your situation. But they are not you. They are looking at the scenario through their own eyes and not yours. Only you can see the question/problem/decision through your lens, so you need to think it through for yourself.

The reality is that the mind which holds the problem, or question, or life decision which needs making, also holds the solution. Go back and read that statement again. The mind may well be so overwhelmed that it can't find the answer at that specific moment, but rest assured the answer is there; it just needs to be teased out.

Your mind has the right solution for you every single time. There is no exception to this. You just need the right tool to access the answers.

This is where calm thinking time is so important.

I have always had a special place in nature which I go to when I want to think something through. The actual place has changed as I have moved around through my life, but I always have a special spot where I can anchor myself. I have found that having a specific place which I can visit when I need to make an important decision has helped me enormously. I will think out loud. I will talk through the situation and all of the possible solutions and I will see which one feels to be the right answer for me. I will sit in silence and see what other ideas spring to mind.

Having specific quiet thinking time allows your mind to calm down and to rest where there are no other interruptions. When your mind is calm, new thoughts can come. You are ready to hear them and can feel if they are right for you. There is just you, nature and your thoughts.

Another option for thinking something through is to think with a friend. However, there are some rules which need to be agreed to in order for you to find the right solution or answer to what you want to think about. The first one is that your friend, the listener, is not allowed to interrupt you whilst you are thinking. When people interrupt us, our brain gets stressed as it hasn't been able to get to the end of its thought pattern. When our brains are stressed, they do not do their best thinking. This may feel counter-intuitive, because during everyday conversations, we always offer our opinions or open our mouths as soon as we think the other person has finished. Sometimes, we have something so important to say that we talk over them. In the case of this calm thinking time though, the only job for the listener is to just listen; listen until the end, offer no advice and no comments. The listener simply lets the thinker think their question or problem through for themselves.

This exercise may feel unusual for you, the thinker, because you are used to friends offering their thoughts and advice to your problems, but persevere and see what happens. You may start thinking out loud by talking the situation through and then your thoughts dry up. If this happens, just sit with the subject for a minute or two and you will be surprised that something new pops into your mind. It's like taking your mind for a walk in the woods. Just talk and see where it leads. It is an extremely powerful exercise.

When doing this exercise with a friend, set a limit for your thinking time; maybe 10 or 15 minutes to begin with. At the end of the time which you have allocated, reverse the roles. The listener now gets their chance to think and the other person takes on the role of the listener.

Both of these thinking techniques whilst in nature or with a friend will help you to find the right solution for you, because it is your mind finding the answers. Both techniques allow you to think calmly which is extremely beneficial for your mental health.

TRY THIS EXERCISE...

Think of something which you would like to think through. Maybe you have a decision to make or you need to decide on a course of action. Make sure that you won't be interrupted. Set an alarm for 15–20 minutes. Talk the topic through out loud to yourself. Talk through the situation and what you believe are the solutions. As you're talking, which option / action feels like it's the right one? If none of them feel right then sit in silence and ask yourself what other options there are. Wait, be patient and see what comes to mind.

SUGGESTED ACTION

- *Find yourself a thinking friend to try the partner technique described above. Review afterwards whether you both found it useful or not.*

- *If you like thinking by yourself, locate yourself a quiet spot in nature where you can go to think quietly.*

Having thinking time helps to manage your mental wellness, particularly when you feel overwhelmed, stressed or when you have an important decision to make.

Mental Well-Being Next Steps

Before you move on to the physical and spiritual well-being sections, take a minute to reflect on what you have read so far.

Review the score which you gave your mental well-being at the beginning of the book. What was it? Where do you want it to be?

What one or two activities have resonated with you the most whilst you were reading this mental well-being section? Write them down. For a summary of all exercises and suggested actions see Appendix two.

What are you going to start putting into practise? Write it down.

If you'd like to get started straight away then turn to section four – Getting Started. Otherwise continue with me to discuss your physical well-being.

SECTION TWO

Physical Well-Being

Why Physical health is so important

We are all spiritual beings having a physical experience here and now on this Earth. Therefore, it is equally important to nourish and look after this vessel or human body which we are currently inhabiting to ensure we stay healthy.

Our physical body is what the outside world sees. It represents who we are and how we are recognised by others. It is our brand if you like. Rightly or wrongly, our physical appearance is often how first impressions are made and, indeed, how we are attracted to our life partners.

I see a lot of pressure these days on all age groups to look and be a certain way.

Teenage girls aspire to look like their idols from photo-shopped images. They pump their lips full of goodness-knows-what, they wear false eyelashes and they tattoo their eyebrows. This is all done in the name of fashion and of 'fitting in.' Amongst new mothers, there is an unwritten society pressure that their bodies should bounce back to their pre-children bodies within a few weeks of giving birth. Even though a woman has spent nine months growing another human being, there is a peer expectation to return to a size 10 or 12 in weeks and not the following nine months post birth. And for those of us who are slightly older, there is also a pressure to continue looking as young as possible whilst aging by banishing those wrinkles and laughter lines which have been picked up on the journey so far by pumping our faces full of Botox or succumbing to plastic surgery.

However, this is not just a female issue. Teenage boys are not exempt from peer pressure. They are self-conscious about facial hair, their height, their weight and whether they are wearing the right branded jeans and trainers to be accepted by their peers. Men also have pressures to have the perfect body, a six pack, to be manly and hairy or to be completely smooth depending on what is in fashion at the time. Should they have facial hair or not? Should they cover the greys or grow old in a distinguished fashion? The evidence of this society pressure can clearly be seen in the growth of men's skincare which has been in double digit growth for years now as men, like women, battle the same pressures of growing old gracefully.

At the end of the day, it is no one else's business what we do or don't do with our physical appearance. My one wish however would be for people to be comfortable in their skin and to enjoy being themselves. Each and every one of us is unique and we do not need to conform or to look a certain way at any point in our lives. We are free to be ourselves and to be the wonderful unique individuals which we are.

There are many ways in which we can increase and naturally improve our physical well-being which I will discuss in this section.

My Physical Well-Being Journey And Steps Which Help Me

My interest in nutrition has been, and continues to be, a journey of education. As a family of five we predominantly enjoyed homemade food and very balanced meals. However, on leaving home and living by myself, I'll be honest, I was guilty of being a convenience queen.

Growing up, I loved Marmite and ate it religiously every day for breakfast, maybe for lunch and always as my perfect hangover cure. Sandwiches were always an easy lunch and I probably had sandwiches for lunch every day at school for 14 years. When I went travelling in my early 20's and was on a budget, it wasn't unheard of for me to have toast for breakfast, sandwiches for lunch and pasta or pizza for dinner, as they were easy, cheap and quick to make. On reflection, having now written this down, my diet in my early twenties was probably not far short of 75% wheat and yeast-based products, not to mention way too many carbohydrates.

Not long after returning from travelling, my body clearly decided enough was enough and I experienced a bad case of eczema all over my arms and legs. Having never suffered with this skin condition as a child or teenager, I was mortified to suddenly develop it in my twenties. Out went the skirts and in came the trousers so that I could cover up this embarrassing condition.

Doctors prescribed steroid creams to manage the situation but this really didn't sit well with me. After much reflection, I concluded that, as I hadn't always had this condition, surely there must be another explanation and reason as to why my body had generated eczema now.

I found a nutritionist and decided to investigate whether she could help me with a solution. My first appointment with her was the first time I heard the term 'leaky gut'. Nowadays the subject of gut health and leaky gut are becoming more widely publicised. However, 25 years ago, without the benefits of Google at my fingertips, there was not much information to read.

A leaky gut occurs when the lining of the intestine becomes damaged and therefore allows toxins and bacteria to leak through the intestine wall and into the blood stream. This foreign substance in the blood can cause skin issues, fatigue, food allergies etc. When the gut is leaky it doesn't produce the enzymes needed for proper digestion and as a result the body can struggle to absorb essential nutrients from food. This in turn can also lead to a weakened immune system.

So, following my diagnosis, I changed my diet completely

for the next two months to whole, unprocessed food. This involved no dairy, no wheat/gluten, no refined sugar, no alcohol and no caffeine. I basically went back to a caveman diet of fresh fruit and vegetables, meat and potatoes. It was difficult at the time, but I wanted so much to have beautiful skin back that it was worth it. I also took probiotics/prebiotics and digestive enzymes to mend my gut, along with other key vitamins and minerals to support my body. (Probiotics are live microorganisms which help to improve and restore the good bacteria in the gut. Prebiotics are specialised plant fibres that act as food for the good bacteria and help to improve the growth and balance of these microorganisms. Digestive enzymes help to break down food so that the body can absorb the nutrients more easily.)

I'll be honest, it wasn't easy. Initially, I lost a lot of weight and then, after a while, my energy returned and I was sleeping so much better.

After two months, once my body had de-toxed, my nutritionist used kinesiology to determine foods which my body either accepted or rejected. Kinesiology is a form of therapy that uses muscle monitoring to look at what could be causing imbalances in the body. It is based on the premise that the body, mind and soul form a whole. When they are balanced, energy flows freely around the body. In the case of food intolerances there will be a disruption in energy flow which kinesiologists can read via a muscle weakness. The muscle testing which they do shows whether a given food maintains energy flow or whether it disrupts energy flow.

The conclusion was that my body was gluten intolerant which, on reflection, wasn't too much of a surprise seeing as I had spent 20 years overdosing on wheat-based products! Luckily for me, this was the only intolerance my body was showing, so dairy and other food groups were perfectly acceptable and I could start to re-introduce them all again slowly.

It took my skin three months to repair itself once my gut was healed and, thankfully, to this day, I have not had a repeat episode.

I am not a nutritionist or a doctor and I am not suggesting that cutting out wheat/gluten from your diet will heal eczema. I am just sharing with you my story of how I discovered and healed my leaky gut. My advice to you would always be to seek professional advice for your individual situation from your doctor or nutritionist.

In my mid-twenties I didn't see the point in cooking just for myself. Cooking wasn't something which I particularly enjoyed and most week-days I was working many hours on my career and simply did not have the energy or inclination to cook when I got home. So, for a number of years, I would happily eat ready meal after ready meal which I threw into the microwave without too much thought. For me, food was a necessity. It was a substance to keep me going. It wasn't something which I really enjoyed and I would much rather have chosen an evening clubbing than an evening at a nice restaurant.

During this time, I started working for a well-known food company. We did a lot of market research to understand the nation's attitude to food and cooking. Cooking from scratch at that time was becoming a lost art due to the rise of good value, convenience food. But the onset of technology and multiple TV channels needing to be filled 24–7 meant the start in the growth of cooking programmes. More recently, these programmes have grown hugely in popularity. There is always a cookery programme of some description on every time you switch on the television and they have probably saved the nation from becoming a pile of unhealthy takeaway slobs!

Just after the millennium, food companies were under pressure to encourage people to cook as well as to educate consumers on healthy mid-week meals. I was involved in many instore marketing campaigns to encourage the nation to cook from scratch and to provide them with some well needed inspiration. Two of the campaigns I managed were 'Roast Britannia' and 'Wake up your Wok'. I'll leave you to work out who I was working for at the time!

What I learnt from my time at this company was how to cook from scratch. We had a team of product developers who spent their days in our large product studios mixing and experimenting with new flavours and concocting new sauces and dishes from around the world. I was lucky enough to have many cookery lessons in these studios and I also learnt a few tricks of the trade. There was never a shortage of volunteers for product tastings and the love of food was clear to see amongst the product designers and employees too. Tasting vindaloo for breakfast however was probably a step too far for me, but it was all part of my job at the time!

However, my awareness of specific ingredients and food came under more scrutiny when I had children. As a new mum weaning a baby for the first time, I read a number of books which all talked about the importance of cooking from scratch and minimising shop-bought alternatives as much as possible. For the first year of my son's life he ate solely home cooked food, including every vegetable known to man and minimal wheat. It was clear to see how much energy he used to have after eating and it felt so good to know that nothing artificial or processed passed his lips, at least in the first year. I congratulated myself on a job well done. However, as a lot of mums reading this will know, this is virtually impossible to commit to unless your sole focus in life is food and planning every meal and snack. So, when I fell pregnant with my second child, I realised that this home cooked food track was unrealistic and I started to allow a few processed foods to join the diet.

In terms of exercise, I have always exercised and found new sports to enjoy and fit into my schedule prior to children. The form of exercise changed over the years as my interests changed and my life took different directions. I did dancing, athletics, badminton, swimming, gym sessions, pilates and yoga. However, the struggle to include exercise in my weekly routine came once I became a mum. I just felt completely exhausted and the idea of exercising was the last thing which I wanted to be doing after the children went to bed. Even when the children were a bit older, finding time to prioritise exercise amongst juggling work, the children and household was always a challenge. It's one area of my well-being which definitely needs more focus.

My interest in skin care products came about when my son developed skin rashes as a young baby. Using prescribed creams did not sit well with me and so I started my investigations into alternative solutions. To be honest what I discovered shocked me. Products from leading baby care brands which I trusted were full of fillers, harsh chemicals and preservatives. They may have smelled amazing but they were full of rubbish and not something which I wanted to be using on my children. I was lucky to be introduced to the Arbonne brand completely by chance by a friend of mine. Arbonne's products are plant-based and completely safe for the whole family. So, for me, this was an easy swap and I've never looked back.

I have always had periods in my life when I suffer with exhaustion. This can be a symptom for so many things that I would always encourage you to talk to your doctor about what could be causing it for you. I have improved my diet, cut out coffee and increased my water consumption. I take a gut health product each day, do at least 15 minutes of movement every day, have periods of rest during my day and go to bed early when I need that extra sleep. Understanding sleep patterns and the types of sleep has helped me to manage my energy levels during different phases. We are changing and growing all of the time, so it's important to know that what works for you today may need adapting tomorrow.

Events have always shown up in my life to point me to a new discovery or a new direction. For example, my diet needed sorting so my body gave me a nudge with the eczema. My son developed a rash which led me to use better body care products. I felt so tired during the day, so I investigated napping and how to re-energise naturally with meditation and periods of rest.

So, I hope that you can benefit from what I have learnt so far on my journey and how to look after your physical well-being with the following chapters.

What Does Physical Well-Being Mean To You?

What is your current physical well-being score out of ten? What would you like it to be?

Are you aware of the areas which you would like to improve?

Do you already know some techniques which work for you?

Signs that you need to focus on your physical well-being include, but are not limited to : tiredness, lethargy or fatigue, being over or underweight, having skin issues, brain fog, health concerns, headaches and migraines and trouble sleeping.

This list is not exclusive. As I explained in the Introduction, well-being strategies are not mutually exclusive. There are other facets of well-being which can help with physical well-being such as positive affirmations and massage (see Appendix one).

Let's discuss some strategies which can help you improve your physical wellness.

1 Nutrition

Probably the biggest influence on our physical well-being is what we eat. We are what we eat. How many times have you heard this? Do you believe it? Is this true for you? Have you really taken the time to sit and think about this statement? Is your relationship with food a healthy one? Do you eat to just fill yourself up or, are you at the other end of the spectrum where you believe that food fuels your soul? These are interesting questions to think about whilst you read this section.

We should think of the human body as a machine. This means, it needs to be fueled regularly in order for it to function correctly and to keep us alive. We can choose to feed it goodness with foods which serve us well and nourish the body or, we can choose empty calories, artificial ingredients and processed offerings. The choice is entirely ours.

Prior to the 1970's the majority of families would have cooked from scratch. However, during the late eighties and nineties, the growth in convenience dishes, microwaveable meals and processed foods in the UK exploded. This was mainly due to the demand from working people who were cash rich but time poor and who were regularly rushing from one place to another without the time to prepare and cook a meal from scratch. Takeaway foods also flourished at this time with the Golden

Arches (McDonald's) springing up on every high street and takeaway Chinese, Indian and pizza just became the norm. It is not really a surprise that when comparing the generation of my childhood to where we are today, there are significantly more weight issues and obesity. The tables have indeed turned since my youth and at the time of writing (2020), it is often cheaper to buy a processed meal than to buy the fresh ingredients and make a meal from scratch. Herein lies the big problem.

It's interesting to think about your own childhood experience with food as you will likely have carried forward these attitudes to food into your adulthood. Did you have a balanced diet? Were your meals home cooked? Were you aware of what you were eating on a daily basis?

Has your awareness of food and what you eat changed over the years? Have you ever stopped to analyse what ingredients are actually in the food which you eat?

There has been a huge resurgence in veganism especially over the last five years. The animal rights movement is obviously a huge reason as to why a lot of people choose veganism. Climate change and the environment is another important factor. Health reasons are also a factor as there is growing research to show the benefits of a diet free from animal products on the human body.

Vegetarian diets are very popular too and there is also growing research on the benefits of choosing this lifestyle. A vegetarian diet has been shown to help heart health by lowering both cholesterol and blood pressure. It can also help you to manage your weight as you cut down on fatty meats and empty calories. However, you also need to manage portion size and not just swap meat for higher calorie foods.

Have you tried being a vegetarian or vegan? If so, what challenges did you face? Did you experience any tangible benefits?

Simply Well-Being

In my experience, the UK is way ahead of other countries when it comes to allergies and diet preferences when eating out. Most restaurants cater for gluten free, dairy free, nut free and vegan diets and indicate accordingly on their menus. My experience in other countries is not so great and I look forward to them catching up very soon.

What Is A Balanced Diet?

A balanced diet is one which contains all of the food groups: carbohydrates, protein, fat, fibre, vitamins and minerals. A nutritious well-balanced diet helps to boost your immune system and keep you healthy.

Are you happy with your current diet? Would you consider your diet healthy ? Is there anything which you would like to change?

Let's have a look at some balanced options:

1. 'Five a Day' of fruit and vegetables is a good rule which we go by in our house. One of my children likes minimal fruit but loves cucumber and carrots whilst the other one will eat pretty much everything apart from sweetcorn. Mix it up a bit. Try the seasonal fruits and vegetables and keep the five a day in your head whilst planning meals.

   Whilst living in Switzerland and shopping there and just over the border in France, I really noticed seasonal fruit and vegetables. The UK tends to have most produce available all year round and, although the strawberries you can buy at Christmas are very expensive, you can still buy them! In Europe it's not the same story. Nectarines and peaches disappear from shelves by the end of August, parsnips and butternut squashes are only available from October to January and the only strawberries available after summer are to be found in the frozen food department. This was all new to me when we moved to Switzerland, but it was good to embrace the produce of the different seasons. For one, it meant that the food was always fresh and local and had not been frozen or shipped half-way around the world to reach our plates, and two, buying local and seasonal produce also helped the planet and kept us healthy at the same time.

As well as your five a day, include some of the following:

- higher fibre foods like potatoes, bread, rice or pasta

- dairy or dairy alternatives (such as almond milk)

- protein such as beans, fish, meat, eggs or pulses.

Choose whole foods over processed ones where possible. Whole foods are higher in important nutrients and tend to be lower in sugar than processed food. Also choose a healthier oil to cook with such as extra virgin olive oil. The main fats in olive oil are monounsaturated fatty acids (MUFAs) which experts consider to be a healthy form of fat.

2. Portion size is another way to achieve a balanced diet. Experts quote this rule of thumb for a healthy plate:

- ½ vegetables and fruit

- ¼ carbohydrates i.e potatoes, pasta, rice

- ¼ protein i.e. fish, meat, eggs.

This is an important one to visualise when you are filling your plate with food.

3. The Food and Nutrition Board also publish guidelines on the Recommended Daily Allowances (RDA) for food groups and vitamins and minerals. These are defined as 'the average daily dietary nutrient intake level sufficient to meet the nutrient requirement of nearly all (97 to 98 percent) healthy individuals in a particular life stage and gender group.'

Recommended Daily Allowance		
	Women	Men
Calories	2,000 kcal	2,500 kcal
Protein	45g	55g
Carbohydrates	230g	300g
Sugars	90g	120g

Eating a diet heavy in meat or carbs just leaves me feeling bloated and sluggish. Perhaps you can relate to that feeling after Christmas when you've eaten and drunk everything without a care in the world, only to awake on New Year's Day definitely a few pounds heavier than when you opened that first door on the advent calendar!

Do you know how your daily diet measures up to the allowances above? Keeping a food diary will show you whether you are consuming too much or too little of one particular food group.

Diets Vs Healthy Living

You can have your pick of the books when it comes to specific diets. For any diet that you can possibly dream up, I am fairly confident there will be a book on it!

The main purpose of most specific diets is predominantly to lose weight. There are some very healthy diet options available and there are also some absurd ones too. I would encourage you to do your research before you get started and to check with your doctor where necessary.

A vast number of these fad diets help you to lose weight, only for you to put the weight back on when you go back to your normal everyday diet. Personally, I believe that the key is to find which foods are serving you and which ones cause you to put on weight. A lot of people are intolerant to some food groups without being consciously aware of this. Intolerances to wheat, gluten, dairy and refined sugar are not uncommon. They can cause bloating, digestion problems, stomach cramps, skin problems, brain fog, headaches and tiredness to name but a few.

Do you have any of these symptoms?

If so, it really is worth identifying whether any of the above food groups are causing you any issues. One way to do this is to cut out all of these processed food groups such as gluten products, dairy, refined sugar and alcohol. After 30 days, you can introduce one food group at a time back into your diet. If you experience any stomachaches, bloating or other symptoms after eating the reintroduced food group, you know that your body has an intolerance to it. Alternatively, you can seek out a nutritionist who can help you identify any food allergies.

Since my early twenties I have followed a gluten-reduced diet. I do not have coeliac disease (where the immune system attacks the body's tissues when exposed to gluten, a protein found in wheat, barley and many other grains) but I do have an intolerance to wheat and feel very unwell if I eat too much of it. Everyone is different but it is worth finding out if you have any food intolerances.

It is also prudent to pay attention to the food which you are purchasing and what it actually contains. The majority of diet-specific food options and processed food contain artificial additives and preservatives. These are usually the list of E numbers on the ingredients list (E numbers replace the chemical or common name of particular food additives. They are used to enhance the colour, flavour or to prevent food from spoiling). In recent years a lot of food manufacturers have ditched specifying the E numbers in favour of long chemical names instead, which are just as confusing for shoppers. These artificial ingredients are exactly that, artificial. Artificial means that our bodies have no idea what to do with them or how to process them. Some of these ingredients pass through our systems whilst the body holds onto others. These artificial ingredients may help to decrease the price of food but there are some considerable health concerns with these types of ingredients. Buying whole, unprocessed food where possible is more beneficial to your health.

Twice a year I do a 30 Days to Healthy Living Programme. It's a re-set which cleanses the body of any toxins which may have been building up over time (a toxin is a poison produced by a living organism such as a plant or animal). It's a very simple programme where all processed foods and food groups which can cause imbalance in the human body are eliminated, including refined sugar, gluten products, dairy, alcohol and soy. It's not a diet, it's a healthy way of eating and living. It includes just pure, whole foods with healthy food supplements which support the body whilst it is detoxing and re-balancing in a healthy way. There are no points to track, no weighing of food or counting calories. I can eat as much as I like providing it is pure, whole food. When the body is free from toxins, it will function more effectively and re-balance naturally at its ideal weight.

Even though I eat pretty healthily most of the time, it's amazing when I do the 30 day programme how much more energised I feel, how I sleep so much better, how clearer my skin is, how clearer my mind is and how I can concentrate for longer.

Are we what we eat? For me, my research is clear – absolutely!

Your Relationship With Food

What is your relationship with food? Is it positive or negative? Do you feel good or bad when you are eating? Or does it differ depending on what you are eating?

For me, this is where the different facets of well-being overlap. Having a positive attitude and mindset towards food has a positive influence on your physical well-being too. Having positive affirmations which relate to food and nutrition is extremely beneficial.

For example:

- I choose to eat healthily every day

- My daily food provides all the nutrients which my body requires

- My diet is healthy and my body thrives

- I nourish my body with healthy, whole food.

Why not write yourself a positive affirmation to help you to achieve your nutrition goal?

TRY THIS EXERCISE...

To aid your physical well-being, take stock of your current diet. Understand if it is balanced, how it leaves you feeling during the day and whether the foods you are eating are serving you or not. Answering the following questions may help you to get started:

- *Are you eating too much sugar, meat, carbs, processed food? Refer to the RDA chart for recommended daily amounts.*

- *Do you feel energised and raring to go after eating or are you ready for a quick siesta on the sofa?*

Another useful exercise is to keep a food diary for a few weeks. Write down everything which you eat including all main meals and snacks etc. Also, write down how you feel an hour after eating:

- Do you feel bloated?

- Do you still feel hungry?

- Do you feel energised or tired?

- What time did you eat?

- How big was the portion size?

Completing a food diary will help you in a number of ways. You will clearly see:

- which foods are helping you feel energized and which foods are making you feel sluggish

- how often you are eating and what the time gap is between meals

- whether you are getting your five a day

- whether you are eating more meat, fish or vegetarian meals

- how many meals you are eating a day

- how many snacks you are eating – is this due to hunger or boredom?

- how many sugary foods you eat or rely on every day for an energy boost

- whether you eat breakfast every day

- whether you are giving your body a rest by leaving a 12 hour gap between dinner and breakfast. (12 hours allows for complete digestion)

Once you have your diary and have analysed what is making you feel good, you can decide on your next steps. As with all things, I would advise making one or two changes at a time. For most people, moving from being an avid carnivore to being vegan overnight is just not a realistic goal or certainly not sustainable in the long term. Choosing to add another vegetarian meal to your weekly menu however is very achievable. Choosing to have your five a day and keeping yourself accountable to this for 30 days is, again, very achievable and a great daily habit.

You decide what is right for you. Where can you make improvements to help improve your daily nutritional well-being?

SUGGESTED ACTION:

- *Keep a food diary.*
- *Add another vegetarian meal to your week.*
- *Add a vegan meal to your week.*
- *Add another fish dish to your week.*
- *Commit to your five a day for 30 days.*
- *Just one sweet snack per day.*
- *Eat breakfast daily.*
- *Keep a 12-hour window before dinner and breakfast for 30 days.*

Choose what your new nutrition goal is going to be, write it down and stick to it for 30 days. Review how you feel.

2 The Importance of Drinking Water

Water – H2O – a clear liquid which freezes at zero degrees and boils at 100 degrees Celsius. It is a simple, unassuming substance, one which many of us take for granted and yet it is a daily necessity for our survival. It became clear to me on researching this topic that we could all do with taking some time to really think about water, whether we consume enough and whether we take it for granted.

We should be appreciating this everyday liquid and giving thanks for it every day, as without it we could not survive for very long at all. For many in the western world, water is taken for granted. It is a commodity which is readily and always available. However, we must remember that this is not the case in all parts of the world. Many people have to walk for miles a day to collect and carry water back to their homes. Millions still live without access to daily clean water. So, for those with clear running water at their disposal every time they turn their taps, perhaps some daily gratitude or thanks could be voiced? How different would your life be if this wasn't the case?

"If there is magic on this planet
it is contained in water"

LOREN EISELEY (1907–1977)
ANTHROPOLOGIST AND NATURAL SCIENCE WRITER

So why do we need water? The adult human body is made up of over 60% of water. Children and teenagers are composed of an even higher percentage. When we look at the key organs which keep us alive, they too are composed of a high percentage of water:

According to H.H. Mitchell, Journal of Biological Chemistry 158, the brain and heart are composed of 73% water, and the lungs are about 83% water. The skin contains 64% water, muscles and kidneys are 79%, and even the bones are watery: 31%.

These percentages blew my mind when I started my research. This information alone of how important water is to our vital organs should have us all running to the tap to drink more water without any further explanation! However, statistics show that half of adults do not drink enough water and some admit to not drinking any water at all on a daily basis. How can we expect our bodies and organs to function effectively and efficiently if we aren't providing them with enough water?

Let's look at the issues which can arise if we don't drink enough water.

Being dehydrated has many negative effects on the body and the mind, for example, dry skin, constipation, a lack of energy, not being able to think clearly and frequent headaches, to name but a few. Drinking enough water really is fundamental to our overall physical and mental well-being. It is widely known that when you feel thirsty your body is already dehydrated and you should replenish your water levels straight away. Take a moment to reflect right now, how many times a day do you feel thirsty?

Also, without sufficient water in our diet, our elimination organs (liver and kidneys) can struggle to do their job properly and as a result toxins can build up in our systems. The human body also tries to hold onto the water which it does have and this in turn can cause the body to put on weight.

As a child, my grandmother would always ask for a cup of hot water after dinner, not tea or coffee, but a hot water. I thought this was a strange thing to drink and when I asked her about it, her response was that she'd been told that she needed to increase her water intake and this was one way to achieve it. She was used to drinking tea after dinner, so switching to hot water was a quick win for her.

I was introduced to a fascinating book in my early twenties which talks about the healing properties of water and the benefits of drinking enough water daily to help prevent illness in our bodies. I would encourage you to look it up and take a read:

Your Body's Many Cries for Water – A Revolutionary Natural Way to Prevent Illness and Restore Good Health. By Dr F Batmanghelidj

Dr Batmanghelidj was best known for his belief that drinking water and increasing water consumption could cure disease.

You may not agree with everything which Dr Batmanghelidj states in his book about water, but it definitely gives food for thought (so to speak!). A lot of aches and pains in our body could be because we are not providing our bodies with the necessary fluids for them to function properly.

Physical Well-Being

If we drank enough water, then:

- our brains would have enough to help us think more clearly
- our kidneys and livers could flush through all the toxins
- our bodies could generate our blood more effectively.

And in turn we would benefit from:

- clearer skin
- efficient muscles and joints
- clear thinking
- more energy
- weight loss
- improved sleep.

For me, the benefits of drinking sufficient water daily are clear. However, we need to make a conscious commitment to increase our water intake on a daily basis to help improve our well-being. This increase should not be liquids in general but just pure water, so that the body does not have to do any work in breaking it down.

What liquids have you consumed so far today?
Write a list.

How many drinks did you have yesterday?
Can you write a list and remember everything
which you drank yesterday?

How many glasses of water do you typically have in
one day?

This is an interesting exercise to do. Are you happy with your drinks list? Do you think that you are drinking enough water?

So How Much Water Should You Be Drinking Daily?

This is a question with many possible answers. Some experts state that adults should drink one and a half litres of water a day. Others say two litres. Some say it depends on the size, weight and mass of a person. Others say it depends on a person's metabolism and that there is not one size which fits all. It will also depend on how active a person is and how much exercise they do as this too will affect the optimum amount of water which needs to be drunk daily. So, I cannot give you a definitive quantity of water to drink to ensure your body is working at its optimum performance. However, I think that most scientists and doctors are in agreement that around six eight ounce glasses of water, or one and a half litres, a day is a good optimal amount to aim for, in addition to all of the other drinks which you are consuming daily.

If you don't currently drink any water at all this might seem like a huge volume of water to consume. I would suggest that you start with a commitment to yourself to just increase your daily drinking by a glass a day and aim to build this up over a number of days to a minimum of four to six glasses of water every day. Alternatively, you could choose to invest in a one and a half litre bottle of water which you fill every morning and slowly work your way through it during the day.

Depending on your lifestyle and daily activity you may need to adjust this quantity. Of course, consumption of other liquids is essential on top as well. I personally find it easier to consume my water intake during the week when I'm working at my desk and can have a pint glass of water by my side as a constant reminder to drink. Or I fill my one litre water bottle and make sure that I've finished one by lunchtime and one by the evening. For me, the weekends prove trickier when I'm busy with the family and I'm out and about. Having a bottle of water with you at all times acts as a good reminder and helps you to drink more.

You need to find what works for you. Take the cue from yourself, tune into how you are feeling and how often you feel thirsty. As with creating all new habits, make a plan, write it down, include it on your weekly to do list and find a way to make drinking water a priority. Some options could include:

- having a glass of water before every cup of tea or coffee.

- starting each morning with a cup of hot water and a squeeze of lemon.

- putting a Post-It note on your bathroom mirror to remind yourself to have a glass of water every time you use the bathroom.

- carrying a bottle of water with you at all times.

Simply Well-Being

Whatever works for you, get creative on daily reminders.

Try an increase in drinking water for 30 days, i.e. 3–4 extra glasses a day. Write down at the beginning how you are feeling, take a photo of your skin, and consider on a scale of one to ten how able you are to concentrate. Do you easily get distracted? Do you frequently feel thirsty? Answer the same questions after two weeks and then again at the end of the 30 days. What benefits have you experienced? Have you noticed any changes in your skin, energy levels or concentration levels? Being aware of the benefits and experiencing them for yourself will mean that you are far more likely to keep this new habit than to slip back into old ways.

Once consuming water switches from a conscious goal to a daily habit, you will have created a positive change to your well-being.

SUGGESTED ACTION

Increase daily water intake – this will depend on how much you drink currently:

- *additional one litre a day.*

- *additional one and a half litres a day.*

- *additional two litres a day.*

- *start each day with a cup of hot water and lemon.*

- *drink a glass of water before every tea and coffee.*

3 Gut Health

How is your gut health? Have you given it much consideration up to this point?

Here are some questions to help you to assess the health of your gut:

- Do you feel bloated after eating?

- Do you suffer with Irritable Bowel Syndrome (IBS)? (IBS affects the large intestine with symptoms including cramping, abdominal pain, bloating and gas.)

- Do you suffer with diarrhoea or constipation?

- Do you open your bowels daily or is it days between movements?

- Is your skin clear or do you suffer with any skin condition?

- Have you recently taken anti-biotics? (Anti-biotics can have negative effects in the gut as they can kill healthy gut bacteria. Taking pre/probiotics after a course of anti-biotics helps to restore the gut to a healthy state).

- Do you suffer with headaches and fatigue?

Some medical professionals accept the importance of gut health on our overall well-being whereas others are yet to be convinced. Research into leaky guts is only just beginning to scratch the surface in this area, so I would urge you to do your own research particularly amongst holistic practitioners, nutritionists and dieticians. These practitioners understand how important our gut health is and that it is our gut which is known to balance our immune system.

If you're stressed out, physically out of balance, run down, recovering from illness or taking anti-biotics, your gut may not be functioning efficiently and you may not be getting all the nutrients from your food to help to build your immune system back up.

Put simply, your intestines are full of bacteria, good and bad. However, you need more good bacteria to keep the bad at bay, to keep your digestion flowing and to keep you looking and feeling healthy. To maintain your gut in a balanced state, a daily dose of prebiotics, probiotics and digestive enzymes is ideal to keep you healthy on the inside. Pro/prebiotics keep the good bacteria growing in the gut and digestive enzymes help your body to break down the food and absorb all of the nutrients easily. If your gut is healthy, then your body functions efficiently and effectively and ultimately you feel healthier.

It has also been proven that your gut produces the good feeling hormone serotonin which can improve your mood. Serotonin is a neurotransmitter or chemical messenger in the body. It is sometimes known as the happy chemical as it has been proven to play an important part in regulating moods and contributes to feelings of happiness. Serotonin is primarily found in the gut and also plays a role in controlling cardiovascular function, bladder control and bowel movements.

According to research studies, serotonin plays a vital role in the communication between your gut and your brain as well as the proper functioning of the gut. It is the gut bacteria which manufactures around 90% of the body's serotonin. So, this again reiterates the importance of your gut health on your overall well-being.

A healthy gut is not only key to a healthy digestive system

but also a key contributing factor to your overall physical well-being.

There is a multitude of prebiotics and probiotics in the marketplace. I recommend that you seek the guidance of a professional nutritionist/dietician for a recommendation. I have found a brand which is clean, toxic free and vegan which specialises in many nutritional and health products. The brand is called Arbonne and I take the Gut Health product daily. All the ingredients promote healthy gut bacteria and a good healthy digestive system.

You can also support your gut health through your diet. Eat foods which are high in fibre, such as fruits and vegetables, beans and legumes as these promote the growth of healthy gut bacteria. Healthy fats, lean meats and cultured dairy products such as live yoghurts, are also good for a healthy gut. Avoid processed and refined junk foods.

A leaky gut can take anywhere from four weeks to six months to repair itself. The condition does not manifest overnight, therefore it will take a while to heal. You will know when your gut is healing when your energy and vitality return. Other healing signs are when you have daily bowel movements, you have no bloating, your mood has improved, you can think clearly and you feel like yourself again.

SUGGESTED ACTION

- *Keep a diary of how you feel when you eat certain foods. Do they make you feel bloated? Do they make you feel energized?*
- *Take a recommended pro/prebiotic and digestive enzyme for 30 days and record how you feel at the beginning and the end of the time period.*

4 Skin Products

Our skin is the largest organ in the human body. It is responsible for guarding our muscles, bones, ligaments and all our internal organs. Our skin and, more specifically our face, is 100% of our 'selfie' and the part which we show to the world every day. Its function is to protect us and to act as a barrier to bacteria, chemicals and variations in temperature.

When we sit and consider all of the functions of the skin listed above and realise what a large part of our visible being the skin represents, don't you think that we should spend more time caring for it, nurturing it and understanding what we are putting on it each and every day? When it comes to healthy living and physical well-being, what we put on our skin is just as important as what we put into our bodies.

The skin is a porous substance, which means that anything which we put onto our skin is absorbed and makes its way into our body, blood and lymphatic system. Research has shown that the level of absorption varies depending on the area of skin in question. For example, our facial skin is more absorbent than our back and our under arm is the most absorbent of all areas. Studies also show that anything between 64% and 100% of substances and fragrances are absorbed by the skin and ultimately make their way into the body.

With this in mind, I believe it is therefore so important to pay attention to the ingredients in our body care, skin care and make-up products including all wash-off products too such as soaps, body washes and hair products. Although these latter products are rinsed off, their ingredients and fragrances can still be absorbed by the skin whilst we are in the bath or shower. Don't be fooled into thinking that if a product is for sale on a retailer's shelf, then it must be 'safe'. There is currently an EU list of around 1,400 ingredients which are banned from skin care and body care products but there are also a lot of chemicals, preservatives, allergens and irritants which aren't included on this list which may well be in the products you use daily.

I'm not advocating for us all to become qualified chemists overnight so that we can understand the ingredient list on the back of our products. However, what I am recommending is that you exercise due diligence. Conduct your own research and find yourself a brand which is open, honest and transparent about its ingredients and where they come from. You may well find a label which states '98% Natural' and think "Great, that's for me!" However, that product could have 2% of harsh chemicals. Also, a word of warning about the word 'natural'. If you see a product which states that it is 100% natural, the perception could be that this is a good brand with no nasty ingredients. But this may not be the case at all. Petroleum jelly is a natural product (a byproduct of crude oil) but you wouldn't want to rub it all over your skin, would you? At least, I hope you wouldn't!

Stop for a minute and add up how many personal care products you use each day. Do you know what is in all of these products?

There are a number of side effects of poor-quality skin care, body care and make-up products which include:

- allergic reactions such as rashes
- dry, flaky, dull skin

- clogging pores which lead to spot breakouts
- redness and sensitivity
- itchiness and stinging.

Do you have any of the above conditions? Could they be caused by any of the products which you are using?

Ingredients To Avoid

Like the growth of processed and convenience food over the last 40 years, the growth in skin care and personal care products has also escalated to mass production. This inevitably means cheap ingredients in order to fulfil the supply chain costs and still provide an affordable product for the end consumer. Manufacturers use cheap fillers to bulk out skin care products which in turn helps to keep the cost low. Mineral oil is one such ingredient which is often added in various guises to skin care products and which is a chemical substance made from naturally occurring crude petroleum oil. Look for ingredients such as petrolatum, paraffinum liquidum, microcrystalline wax, paraffin and synthetic wax to name but a few. Ingredients are listed in order of their volume, so the first ingredient makes up the highest percentage of that product. In a lot of skin care and body care products, you may find that mineral oil is listed as one of the first four ingredients.

Sodium lauryl sulfate (SLS) is an ingredient which is found in many everyday washing and bathing products as it lathers up to create bubbles. Over the years we have been conditioned to believe that we need bubbles in order for a product to clean our hair, body or skin, whereas in reality this isn't true. Although deemed safe to use by many regulatory bodies, SLS has also been proven to irritate skin if left on for too long in some instances.

Manufacturers are required to prove that products are stable for a considerable length of time before they are listed for sale, which means only one thing: the use of preservatives. Formulations need to be stable, fragrances need to be as strong as the day of manufacture when you open the bottle and colours need to remain vibrant throughout the product lifecycle too. Therefore, another ingredient group to look out for is parabens. Parabens is a group of chemicals used as artificial preservatives in cosmetic and body care products. Parabens can disrupt hormones in the body and also cause skin irritation. A lot of brands now state on the front of their packaging whether they are paraben free, as this group of chemicals received a lot of bad press a few years back.

So, whilst TV campaigns may well portray product exclusivity in a bid to get you to buy their brand, the products are mass produced all the same. And, with mass production comes cheap ingredients and shortcuts which are not always in the consumers' best interest.

Find yourself a brand which can explain the purpose of all the ingredients that they have included in their formulations, for example, a brand which advocates only clean ingredients and which has the health of their consumer at the heart of everything which they do. By clean ingredients I mean those which are free of harmful chemicals.

I have found my brand (Arbonne). I know that every product they produce is vegan and certified clean. I know that the ingredients used are of the highest quality and all are sustainably sourced. I know that this company does not allow over 2,000 banned ingredients in any of their products (the EU currently only bans around 1,400 ingredients) and I know that they do not use any ingredient unless it adds value to the product and needs to be there. I am happy that this brand is safe for my family, safe for me and I'm also happy that by using these products I am helping to support a healthy lifestyle and healthy skin.

TRY THIS EXERCISE...

Write down all the products which you use on your body daily. Include all shower, wash, body, shave, make-up, perfume products.

SUGGESTED ACTION:

- *Audit what products you are using. Do they contain any harmful ingredients? Do you know what the ingredients are?*

- *Swap one or two of your daily products to a healthier brand.*

.

5 Exercise

I'm not going to lie, this chapter has been the most challenging to write, as exercise is something which I have always struggled to get excited about! I have not struggled to do exercise, but I do struggle to enjoy it, to be motivated and to keep it as part of my daily and weekly routine. Some of you reading this may well experience a real buzz and an endorphin high after exercising but I've never really experienced this.

What are your thoughts towards exercise? Have you found a sport which you love? Do you regularly schedule exercise into your weekly routine? Or do you struggle to stay motivated and consistent? What would you like your relationship with exercise to be?

As a child I was fairly active. I went to dance classes twice a week, swam and did gymnastics at school. On moving to grammar school, I was on the netball team and athletics team. As I explained earlier in the book, I also played badminton for a local club, which was great cardio exercise. So, I've always been fairly active and tried a number of sports but, unlike other people I know, I've never been one to jump out of bed and do a workout before going to work.

Let's look at why exercise is so important for your physical and your mental well-being.

The benefits of exercising regularly are clear. Not only does exercise keep you fit and in shape, but it has also been proven to be good for your mental health. Your body releases serotonin and endorphins whilst exercising and it is these chemicals which play an important part in regulating your moods. Exercise benefits include:

- helping to manage weight
- strengthening bones and muscles
- lowering blood pressure and improving heart health
- reducing the risk of disease
- improving brain function and memory
- boosting mood and helping to reduce the symptoms of depression and anxiety
- decreasing stress
- increasing self-esteem and self-confidence
- aiding better sleep.

So, how much exercise should you be aiming for? There is no 'one size fits all' when it comes to exercise. It very much depends on you the individual, your health, weight, age and fitness level. It will also depend on what your end goal is. Is it to be fitter? Is it weight loss? Is it body toning? Is it improved mental well-being? A qualified personal trainer will be able to help with a tailored programme for you depending on your goal.

Experts have differing advice on how much exercise is the right amount. Three periods of 30 minutes cardio per week is recommended by some. 10,000 steps a day is another target frequently discussed. Two cardio workouts and some stretching is advised by others. You choose what is right for you. If you currently don't do much exercise at all then a good goal to start with – and one which I live by – is a minimum of 15 minutes of movement per day.

Finding exercise which works for you and which you enjoy is the most important criteria when it comes to keeping fit. Before moving to Switzerland, I attended a local boxercise circuit class with Stuart, a fabulous trainer. Punching a boxing bag was extremely therapeutic for both my physical and mental health and I rarely missed a week in two years. During the Covid lock down I did online workouts with my daughter to replace her PE lessons and of course we did plenty of dog-walking. Having a dog does mean that I have to get out of the house each day regardless of the weather. I set myself a weekly goal last year of walking with Poppy for at least an hour, five times a week. To begin with, this was to ensure my daily step goal was achieved but, after a few weeks of regular, daily walking I realised that these daily walks were so much more than just the exercise for me. My daily walks also provide me with great thinking time. I love being outdoors in the fresh air, I get to appreciate the wonderful place where I live and it puts me in a good frame of mind for the rest of the day. I now look forward to these walks. They are part of my day and I have created a great daily exercise habit once more.

Finding your ideal exercise may take some time, or you may know instantly what you love to do. You might love running, swimming, walking, working out in the gym by yourself, or you might prefer the rigour and set times of specific classes. You might prefer team sports such as football, netball, rugby or basketball etc. Or you might prefer to mix exercise with breathing and mindfulness and do yoga or Pilates. You might prefer to exercise alone, or you might prefer to go with a friend as this gives you the extra encouragement to get moving. It is worth trying a number of exercise options to find something which really floats your boat. If you enjoy it then you are more likely to stay committed. You might be the kind of person who sticks with the same exercise their entire life. Maybe running is your passion and that's all you love to do, or if you are like me, you might change your exercise of choice depending on the season of your life. What works this year may not work for you in 12 months' time. The key to exercise is to enjoy it. Find something fun because then you will look forward to it and you are less likely to quit.

Once you have found your ideal exercise, the next step is to build it into your daily or weekly schedule. Without scheduling it into your diary, it just won't happen and you'll start to find excuses not to do it. You might not always feel like exercising, but you will always feel better for doing it and for following through on your commitment. If you're new to exercising, then I would recommend building up slowly. Commit to one session a week and stick to it. It is far better to do one activity once a week than nothing at all. Start small and build from there.

Far too many people make a New Year's Resolution to get fit. They join a gym and go full out during the first week attending three, four or even five times. To go from nothing to exercising full out every day is unlikely to be a realistic goal which can be maintained long term. After a week, there will be aches and pains, tiredness and exhaustion and that is when excuses not to continue will flood the mind. Setting yourself up for success is important. Choosing something realistic and achievable and then building frequency over time means that you are more likely to succeed in your exercise goals.

Remember to stretch and cool down too, this will help to ease those post-exercise aches you can experience when you haven't exercised for a long time. Remember, the aim is to keep going, to be consistent with your exercise and not to be in so much pain that you decide not to exercise ever again!

Simply Well-Being

SUGGESTED ACTION

- *Decide on your exercise goal and write it down.*

- *Identify a form of exercise that you enjoy and schedule it into your diary. Commit to completing it once a week / twice a week.*

If you don't know where to start maybe think about movement and steps, for example:

- *Commit to 15minutes of movement each day, i.e. walking, jogging, stretching etc.*

- *Commit to 10,000 steps each day or every other day.*

- *Commit to walking up stairs and not taking any lifts.*

- *Incorporate a mindfulness practice to the weekly schedule such as yoga, Pilates or meditation.*

Keeping an exercise diary to track how you feel after each session both physically and mentally is a good habit. Once you know your exercise goal, write it down in your diary and track how you are measuring against your target. As discussed in 'daily wins', this not only helps you to see your progress it also helps to keep you motivated and ultimately boosts your self-esteem.

6 Let's Talk Rest

The human body was not designed to run on ever-ready batteries. In order to function well, our bodies need rest and proper sleep. So, let's start with the subject of sleep.

Getting enough sleep is extremely important for our day-to-day well-being and is a subject which we rarely give much thought or attention to. Waking up feeling tired and lethargic can mean that our bodies and brains won't function properly during the day. We can struggle at school, at work, have brain fog and have difficulty in making decisions to name but a few side effects of a poor night's rest. As a consequence of waking up tired, people reach for caffeine and strong coffee to get them going in the morning followed by refined sugary snacks and chocolate for an extra energy boost when they start to experience that afternoon slump.

Does any of this sound familiar to you? It's worth stopping for a second and thinking about these questions:

- How do you feel when you wake up in the morning?

- Do you feel rested or do you wake up feeling tired?

- Are you reaching for coffee as you like the taste, or do you need the caffeine to stop yourself feeling so tired?

- Do you feel different at the weekend when you wake to no alarm or when you wake an hour or two later?

- How many hours sleep do you get on average during the week?

- How many hours on average do you get at the weekend? Is there a difference?

- Is there a difference to how you feel physically when you wake during the week or at the weekend?

- Do you regularly feel tired during the day?

From your answers, you can identify if there are any improvements which you could make to your sleep patterns which would benefit both your physical and mental well-being.

It is not uncommon these days for many people to burn the candle at both ends of the day. They are up before sunrise and awake until well after midnight. Research has proven however that this continued lifestyle can take its toll on the physical body after a while as the body is not getting enough time to replenish and heal itself. Our bodies need this sleep time to repair and rebuild. When we switch our conscious minds off, all of those trillions of cells which make up our body work to re-balance themselves and come back to a state of equilibrium. This process takes time and cannot be achieved by the body whilst our conscious mind is in control, i.e. during our waking time.

The benefits of a good night's sleep are clear:

- improves attention and concentration
- gives the body time to repair and re-build

- allows the brain to organise and process all the information which has been taken on during the day

- helps to keep energy levels up so we don't need to snack or overeat the following day.

So, how much is enough sleep? This is the million-dollar question and one which will invoke much discussion and debate amongst many people.

Personally, I've always needed a good eight hours sleep a night. Any less than this for a few consecutive days and I feel tired, lethargic and generally very grumpy. However, I also know many people who can easily get away with five or six hours a night.

How many hours of sleep do you typically need? How many hours do you typically get? The two numbers don't always match!

Like all aspects of well-being, everyone is different. We are all unique and there is no one right answer. So, to aid your daily well-being, I would recommend that you listen to your own body to decide how much sleep you need to get. This may vary from week to week, month to month, depending on how much you've got going on, what you are juggling and how stressed you are feeling. Some weeks you may need eight hours sleep a night. Other weeks you may be feeling a bit more depleted and need nearer nine hours. There is no right or wrong, so listen to your body to feel how much sleep you actually need in order for you to wake feeling rested and able to function clearly and effectively during the day.

I was talking with a mum only this week who was saying how tired she felt. So, I suggested that she go to bed as soon as she's put the children to bed. Although this would mean no evening or time to herself, occasionally it's the sensible thing to do and her body and mind would thank her for it. I'm often asleep not long after my children, especially when my husband is away on business. I love that extra couple of hours sleep and I wake feeling much more rested and happier to start the day.

If you regularly wake up in the morning feeling tired, then make a promise to yourself that you will go to bed extra early that evening. If you've had a busy week work-wise and socially, prioritise some extra sleep time at the weekend. Allow yourself to lay in, turn off all alarms and let your body wake up in its own time. Do you feel more energised when you wake naturally?

There are four main sleep stages which we all go through in one sleep cycle, which can last around 90–120minutes.

Stage One is when we are getting ready for sleep, getting ready to switch off. We close our eyes and start to feel drowsy and our heart rate begins to slow down.

Stage Two is the light sleep stage and where we spend most of our sleep. Our breathing and heart rate slows even further.

Stage Three is where we experience deep sleep and where our brain waves are the slowest in frequency. This is an extremely important phase as it is during this deep sleep that the body repairs itself and replenishes.

Stage Four is the rapid eye movement (REM) stage where our eyes move rapidly behind our closed eyelids. This is the stage of sleep when we are most likely to experience dreams.

Although all stages of sleep are important, it is during stage three, deep sleep, that our body does the most work to repair muscles, tissues and cells in our bodies, as well as releasing growth hormones. The length of a sleep cycle will be different from person to person but on average a cycle lasts 90–120 minutes and should ideally be repeated three to four times a night. Sleeping for less than 90 minutes means that your body has not had the chance to go through all the sleep stages and therefore you may experience feeling groggy and lethargic.

Let's talk about napping for a moment. When my children were small and I was juggling working and childcare, an afternoon nap on a Friday was often a necessity for me. My daughter would have a nap after lunch and I would crawl into bed to do the same. Sometimes I would be out for the count until she woke up. At other times I would be woken by the phone or doorbell and would feel cheated that it had been cut short. However, what I did notice was that sometimes I would wake feeling worse than beforehand. I could feel very disorientated and groggy, so I began to question whether napping was a good thing for me or not.

As explained above, the full sleep cycle is around 90 minutes. If you are woken early from deep sleep then this is when you are likely to feel groggy and even more tired than you did before you napped as your body did not make it through one full cycle of sleep. On the other hand, during a nap of 10–20 minutes you are likely to be experiencing light sleep which is beneficial for an energy boost and an increase in productivity. So, my recommendation for napping during the day is to either nap for 10–20 minutes or at least 90 minutes, as anything in between these periods of time might be counterproductive. What I did find helpful was to set an alarm so that I kept my naps short and no longer than 20 minutes. These naps gave me the energy boost I needed.

Difficulty in sleeping can be problematic for some. Periods of insomnia affect around 10–30% of adults and can be brought on by numerous triggers such as stress, worrying about an upcoming event or occasion, death of a loved one, money worries or a new job. If this happens to you, the first thing to say on this subject is to be kind to yourself. Beating yourself up and lying in bed tossing and turning because you just can't get to sleep is doing the exact opposite of helping you drift off to the land of nod.

If you are experiencing a period of insomnia, you need a strategy to break the cycle. Develop a new nighttime routine including wind-down time which is different somehow to your normal bed routine. Switch your phone and laptop off at least an hour before you are due to go to bed. Have a hot bath or shower, drink a hot drink, read a book, meditate, listen to some calming music and develop a new routine which helps you to calm down and start to relax. Always have a pen and paper beside your bed so that you can write down any thoughts or actions which spring to your mind whilst you are trying to wind down and get to sleep. This helps to park those thoughts and release them to tomorrow so that you can focus on getting some rest and falling asleep. Try some breathing techniques. Breathe in to the count of four and out to the count of four and repeat. Visualise the relaxation flowing down from the top of your head to the tips of your toes. Visualise all of your organs and limbs one by one gently relaxing and letting go.

You can experiment with listening to soothing sounds such as the sound of the sea, a trickling stream, rain, birds singing, dolphins calling or whatever helps you to relax. Try some essential oil. Just a few drops of lavender can evoke the body to start feeling relaxed and sleepy. Visualise yourself sleeping soundly and drifting off to sleep easily every night. Repeat a positive affirmation, "My body receives all the sleep it needs" or "I fall asleep quickly and easily as soon as my head touches my pillow."

Regardless of whether you are asleep or whether you are lying in bed relaxing and concentrating on your breathing,

Simply Well-Being

your body is experiencing rest and this is important. It may not be deep sleep but it is rest from rushing and doing and this is equally as important. Maybe you didn't get your eight hours of sleep but you got five hours and a couple of hours of rest. This is significantly better than a couple of hours of tossing and turning and feeling frustrated that you couldn't sleep. So, be kind to yourself.

For ongoing sleep issues, I would recommend hypnotherapy or spiritual response therapy (see the chapters on these therapies for more information) to understand the potential reason behind the insomnia. These therapies can help identify what has triggered the insomnia and how to break the cycle. They are great at helping to provide a solution for a peaceful night's sleep.

Periods of Rest

Apart from sleep, having periods of rest throughout the day is also extremely beneficial for both your physical and mental well-being. Your mind is processing a huge number of thoughts a day which means that it is important to build in some rest periods and downtime during your day. I have written about meditation in section one and how building a meditation practice into your daily routine can help to quieten the mind and re-instill a feeling of calm and tranquility. One way to achieve a quick period of rest is with a one-minute meditation. One minute might not sound like a particularly long period of time and you might be thinking that not much can be achieved in just 60 seconds, but I would disagree. I believe that everyone can find multiple periods of one minute in their day to just stop and focus on their breathing for 60 seconds. At the end of just 60 seconds you will be amazed at how much calmer and back in control you can feel.

Having a break for a cup of tea, going outside for a walk and some fresh air, daydreaming whilst cooking dinner or listening to music are all examples of rest during the day. Whether it's a rest from thinking or a rest from doing, your body needs both. So, embrace these activities and build more of them into your day. Also, notice how you feel after each of these activities. Do you feel calmer? Do you feel more energised? Do you feel happier?

There is a Zen proverb which says that you should meditate/rest for at least 20 minutes during the day unless you are busy or stressed, in which case you should meditate/rest for at least an hour.

It may sound counter-intuitive but it's true. During stressful, busy periods in our lives we do need more rest, sleep and meditation to help our bodies and our minds to process everything which is going on. Failure to do so can lead to fatigue, illness and anxiety. So how much rest and sleep do you need right now? Perhaps the actions below will help.

SUGGESTED ACTION:

- *Keep a sleep diary for a couple of weeks. Record how easy it was to fall asleep, how many hours sleep you get and how you feel when you wake up in the morning. From this information you can then decide if you need more sleep or rest and whether you need to change your bedtime routine at all.*

Other actions could then include:

- *committing to an extra 30mins of sleep a day.*

- *committing to an extra hour of sleep a day.*

- *committing to not setting an alarm at least once a week.*

- *exercising regularly to aid sleep.*

- *changing your alarm to a gentle sound so you awake feeling happy.*

- *devising a new winding down nighttime routine.*

- *switching off your laptop and phone at least an hour before bedtime.*

- *not drinking any caffeine after 5pm.*

- *incorporating a one-minute meditation into every day.*

Physical Well-Being Next Steps

Before you move on to the spiritual well-being section, take a minute to reflect on what you have read in this section.

Review the score which you gave your physical well-being at the beginning of the book. What was it? Where do you want it to be?

What one or two activities resonated with you the most whilst you were reading this physical well-being section? Write them down. For a summary of all exercises and suggested actions see Appendix two.

What are you going to start putting into practise? Write it down.

If you'd like to get started straight away then turn to section four – Getting Started. Otherwise continue with me to discuss spiritual well-being.

SECTION THREE

Spiritual Well-Being

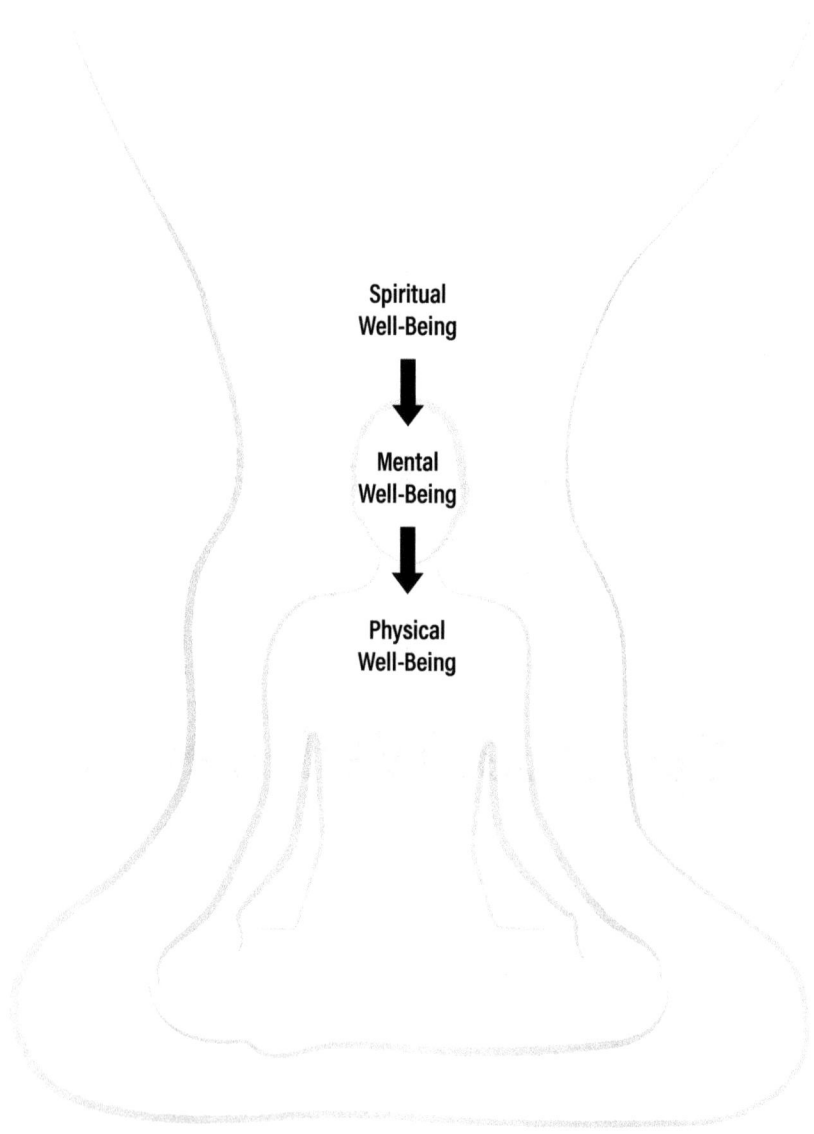

Spiritual
Well-Being

⬇

Mental
Well-Being

⬇

Physical
Well-Being

Three facets of well-being – spirit, mind, body

Why Spiritual health is so important

For me, a book on well-being is not complete without a section dedicated to our spiritual and emotional well-being as, fundamentally, this is the core of who we truly are. We are all spiritual beings in a physical body and therefore it is right that we spend an equal amount of time understanding our spiritual side, nurturing it and ensuring that we are also experiencing spiritual well-being. During my well-being journey I never found a book which included spiritual well-being and yet this is the overarching essence of who we are.

For some of you, this may be a new way of thinking, but for me it is fundamental. As humans we are all mind, body and spirit. The three elements are intertwined and they are not mutually exclusive. Understanding and being aware of all three facets will help to improve your overall well-being no end. When we really examine the subject of well-being, all three areas overlap and influence each other. For example, the food, nutrition and water which we consume not only helps our physical well-being but also our mind's health in terms of being able to think clearly. Also, the meditation exercises which we covered in the mental well-being section not only help our mental health but they are also the gateway to our spiritual side and our higher self (see Appendix One for connected activities). All three areas of well-being are not mutually exclusive, they influence each other and are woven together. Being in tune with your inner peace and your inner being is in essence being in tune with your spiritual higher self.

For our true overall well-being it is important to be balanced and focused on all aspects of ourselves, our mind, our body and our spirit.

Spiritual wellness for you, may or may not include religion. This is a personal choice and one which only you can make.

Religion is not something which I have included in my book. It is too wide a subject to do it any justice here and is personal to everyone. So, I will leave the subject of religion and prayer to your own decision. However, having an understanding that you are connected to something larger than yourself, whatever that means to you, has been proven to help your overall spiritual and mental well-being.

In this section, I will talk about purpose as well as holistic and spiritual healing techniques. Illness can present itself in the body as a result of negative energy, negative thoughts or negative emotions which we have experienced in some area or another. The word disease explains it well. 'Dis' and 'ease', mean lack of ease somewhere in the body. If not released from a spiritual point of view, the negative energy or emotion can ultimately show up at a physical level within the body. Therefore, when you experience any physical symptoms, it is important to not only treat these symptoms but also to treat the mental and spiritual aspects as well. This is where energy healing, reiki healing, hypnotherapy, spiritual response therapy (SRT) and other alternative therapies come into play. All therapies can be used as a preventative measure, to keep your spiritual wellness intact, as well as to help heal existing conditions.

There are a multitude of techniques and I do not confess to know them all. So, I will cover what I personally know in the next few chapters and those techniques which have worked and continue to work for me. As human beings we are all different, we are all unique and, as I have said before in this book, there is not one size which fits all. Your journey will be different from mine. You need to discover for yourself what sits well with your values and your beliefs and what techniques work for you and help you to feel connected and to feel good. This is the one rule which you need to remember each time you try something new or experience something new. Did it, or does it, feel good to you? If it does, great. If it does not, then move on to something else. Always trust your instincts and find out what works for you.

One final thing to bear in mind is that any activity which makes you feel happy and at peace is an opportunity to improve your spiritual wellness.

My Spiritual Well-Being Journey And Steps Which Help Me.

My first recollection of a spiritual event was when I was around seven years old. I shared a room with my sister at the time and I remember lying in bed one evening struggling to sleep. I just lay there staring into the darkness and this voice sounded in my head, "Why am I?" It was a strange question for a seven-year-old to ask, but the more I asked it in my head, the louder the voice became and the more out of my body I felt. The voice and my body felt separate in a way; connected, but separate at the same time. I couldn't quite understand why I was seeing through these eyes of mine. Why was I here in this physical body and not another one? Why was I here right now in this place, in this bed, in this house? Whilst asking these questions, I had a strong knowing that I was part of something larger and that this physical earth was not all that existed.

I got a strong sense that my voice or spirit wasn't tied to this seven-year-old body, it just happened to be in my body at this particular time. I also had the sense that there was more to the world than just being in this young body in my bed in this house.

I couldn't quite intellectualise this as a seven-year-old but years later, when reflecting on the experience, I was able to understand it better. I didn't feel scared. I felt very calm and in control and inquisitive. Why am I? Why am I?

I had this same experience a number of times over the following few weeks. I didn't have a clear answer as to what I was part of but I grew to just know that there was something else to this world. I remember feeling quite calm and reassured. It was almost like there was something which I should be remembering but I couldn't quite put my finger on it at that time.

That was my first recollection of realising that I was part of this huge universe. I didn't know any more than that and I soon forgot all about it until many years later.

I was brought up in a Christian household. My Mother had joined our local Holy Trinity church when we moved house and, on most Sundays, I would accompany her to church with my younger sister. Through these Christian teachings I always believed in the afterlife and would often talk to my grandparents who had passed over. My father on the other hand had other ideas about religion, not that he ever said any religion was categorically wrong, but he had what I considered then to be very alternative views. He would talk about spirituality and Buddhism amongst others. To be honest, I was a typical teenager and never really listened to a word he was saying. My eyes would glaze over and I would think, "Here Dad goes again!".

I was introduced to hypnotherapy when I was 19 years old. Having left school after A-levels and launched into the outside world, I quickly realised that I was ill-equipped to deal with the realities of the outside world and this is when my panic attacks began. After what seemed like an endless period of time and confusion, my mum suggested that I visit a hypnotherapist to see if she could help me.

Up until this point in my life, my only knowledge of

hypnosis was what I had seen sensationalised on television, where willing volunteers were hypnotised and asked to act in ridiculous ways in order to entertain the mass public. I was skeptical to say the least as to how it could help me with my situation. But I was open minded and I had also heard more positive stories that certain hypnotherapy techniques could help people to stop smoking, so I decided that I had nothing to lose.

Hypnotherapy helped me through this difficult time and still does to this day. I was so fascinated as to how it worked that I trained as a hypnotherapist myself, so that I could learn further and help other people.

In my early twenties, I was introduced to spiritual healing through my parents, who both trained with the National Federation of Spiritual Healers (NFSH) in the UK. They volunteered at a Healing Centre in our home town and I was asked to front the reception desk on a Saturday morning, which I did for a couple of years. It was a drop-in centre. No appointment was required, and we would have a steady stream of clients who would stop by for some healing and company. The group of healers who attended the centre were all quite diverse in terms of age, background and experience. I was fascinated with their stories and how they had found spiritual healing. I was repeatedly told that I too was a healer and could also do this type of work but I never completely understood what they meant and at that time I didn't feel that I possessed any talents in this area at all.

However, after a few years intrigue got the better of me and I found myself booked on the Level One course with the National Federation. I wanted to experience first-hand what spiritual healing was all about and whether I was a healer or not.

I remember arriving at the course, looking around and thinking how different I was to everyone else. For a start, I was the youngest person there by far and when we all introduced ourselves to the group, my lifestyle and life stage were also completely different. On day one, I was very unsure that I was in the right place at all. I had huge self-doubt and spent the day constantly worrying what everyone else was thinking of me. I couldn't relax during the meditations and I couldn't feel any energy when working with my hands. It felt very much like I was a fraud, just going through the motions and hoping not to get found out. True 'Imposter Syndrome' was at work!

On day two however, I had an epiphany. One of the ladies was giving me healing as I sat in a chair. I was focusing on my breathing and just listening to the healing music which was being played in the background. I was also pondering a dilemma which I had going on in my life and, if truth be known, I was looking for an answer. Out of nowhere I experienced a heat in my chest right by the heart. That's where it started and from there it spread throughout my torso and all the way up to my face and my head. I had never experienced anything like it before. It was such a lovely energy, calm, loving and healing. I remember receiving an instant clarity of thought on the subject I had been pondering. It was clear. The answer felt good, I felt good and I just knew that it was the right course of action which I needed to take.

In that moment, I knew I was in the right place. I knew I was part of this huge universe and I also knew that I was being looked after by the spiritual world and that it was there to help me on my life's journey. It was an incredible experience and not one which I have shared with anyone until writing this book.

Then it was my turn to reciprocate and to channel healing to this lady. I closed my eyes and asked my spirit guides to help this lady. There were two ways of giving the energy healing which we were learning:

Simply Well-Being

- working within the aura to feel the energy through our hands at the key chakra points (the aura is the energy field around the body and chakras are the main energy centres of the body), or

- by placing our hands on the person where we felt guided to place them.

Up until this point, I had not felt anything when going through the motions the day before. However, during this session my hands felt on fire. I could instantly feel the energy of the chakras as I placed my hands a few inches away from her body. I could also feel if I needed to stay in a certain place for longer and I knew when to move away. The difference was incredible. Personally, I wasn't doing anything differently, but I could feel the energy and I was able to interpret the energy and move my hands to where I was being directed.

I realised that by tuning in, by asking my angels and guides for help and by moving myself out of the equation, that I became a human vehicle through which the energy and healing could flow to my client. I just had to get out of the way. This training day just blew me away! Not only had I experienced spiritual healing directly for myself, but I had also been able to feel the energy and be the vehicle for someone else to experience it too.

Over the next few years, I completed all levels of spiritual healing with the UK NFSH as well as Reiki healing and Indian head massage. I also worked at a similar drop-in healing centre just outside of Windsor. I loved my time there. I met some wonderful people and it was very rewarding work, which was completely different from my corporate day job at the time. That was when I realised that I liked helping people and it would be great if I could find a way somehow to turn this into a full-time career.

What Does Spiritual Well-Being Mean To You?

What is your current spiritual well-being score out of ten? What would you like it to be?

Does spiritual well-being include religion or prayer for you?

Are you aware of the areas which you would like to improve?

Do you already know some techniques or therapies which work for you?

Signs that you need to focus on your spiritual well-being include, but are not limited to: lacking in purpose or direction, feeling lost and disconnected from your environment, experiencing illness, feeling unhappy or unmotivated, having phobias or irrational fears.

This list is not exclusive. As I explained in the introduction, well-being strategies are not mutually exclusive. There are other facets of well-being which can help with spiritual well-being such as meditation, exercise and talking with a friend (see Appendix one).

Let's discuss some strategies which can help you improve your spiritual wellness.

1 Finding Purpose

What gets you out of bed every morning? What do you love doing? How would you spend your time if money was no object? What energises you? What makes you feel alive and happy?

Purpose is an important consideration when discussing well-being as without a purpose or reason to get out of bed each day, low mood, depression and other mental health illnesses may follow.

The definition of Life Purpose is having set goals and a direction in one's life.

Do you know your life purpose? Do you connect with your purpose every day? Do you currently have goals which you are working towards?

These are all good questions to ask yourself as we review purpose and it is absolutely okay if you have answered 'no' to any of the above questions.

I believe that there are multi layers when talking about purpose:

1. Life purpose – long term

2. Direction – medium term

3. Goals – short term

All are equally as important. One of the issues which people can have when they think about life purpose however, is that it sounds so enormous and so critical. It sounds like it is the pinnacle of everything and, as a result, it can paralyse people and stop them from moving forward. People can feel overwhelmed and extremely anxious in case they get their life purpose wrong.

If this is you, then I am here to tell you that it's OK if you don't know your life purpose. Be easy on yourself. I will discuss life purpose and share some ideas with you, but it is more important for you to just find purpose in what you are doing right now. Having a purpose for your day, however big or small that may be. Setting yourself some goals for the short term so that you are working towards something, whether that is a work goal, a well-being goal or a personal goal. This level of purpose where we have goals is what provides us with the motivation and focus on a daily and weekly basis. This is what gets us out of bed each day.

Purpose can be connected to a multitude of areas. For some people, it is connected to their vocation and having meaningful rewarding work. Others find meaning through spiritual and religious beliefs. For others, their purpose lies in their responsibilities to their family or friends. Or purpose can be expressed in all these aspects of life.

Many books have been written on the meaning of life and finding a purpose. Having a reason to get out of bed each day is so important for how you are feeling about your life. Many books on happiness conclude that those people who are truly happy have identified what they love doing and are pursuing their life on purpose. They know what they want to achieve, and when they do something which they love, and which has meaning in their life, then each day is just joyful.

There are many benefits cited for having and knowing your purpose, for example:

- increased optimism
- increased resilience
- increased motivation
- living a more contented and fulfilled life
- experiencing happiness and joy
- ultimately feeling happy.

1 Life Purpose

Life purpose is an underlying theme or goal which encompasses your whole life journey. It is not one specific vocation which you need to find, or one specific goal which you need to achieve. A life purpose or higher purpose runs through your overall life goals and daily goals. It may be something which you are aware of, or you may not have pieced it all together yet. Either is absolutely fine, there is no right and wrong way.

For example, maybe your life purpose is to serve others. As you can see, this 'to serve' is a very specific purpose, however it could be played out in a multitude of ways. There are numerous roles and jobs which fit under this overall purpose e.g. doctor, lawyer, politician, nurse, teacher, fire person, coffee barista, retailer, therapist, customer service advisor, religious leader, financial advisor, social worker, delivery driver or refuse collector. All of these vocations are serving people, but the actual day-to-day jobs and tasks are very different. Outside pursuits and hobbies which fit under this overall purpose could include examples such as team sport coach, volunteering in the community or running a club.

If this is your life purpose, then you could move quite happily from one activity to another as they all have the same common goal of serving others. So, there is not just one job which you are looking for when you think about your overall life purpose. Everyone will have their own interpretation of their life purpose and what activities feel good and are right for them. When you view life purpose as an overarching theme in your life, then it is less scary and allows you the freedom to choose different directions and different executions under this theme. You really can't get it wrong.

Some examples of life purpose could be:

- serving others

- giving back to your community

- fighting for a social cause e.g. animal survival, climate change

- building a business and leaving a legacy i.e. something that makes a difference in people's lives around the world.

- to love and support family, friends and all your connections.

Do any of these resonate with you? By looking back at jobs which you have had or hobbies which you did or are doing, is there any common theme? Which ones have given you the most satisfaction? Can you relate these to a common purpose?

2 Direction

We may not be completely sure what our overall life purpose is. However, having a direction in terms of where we are moving to is also important to us feeling happy and motivated.

When I talk about direction, I mean having a medium-term plan and something which you are working towards. Career-wise, this can mean maybe having a job which you want to be doing in 10 years' time and having a plan as to how you are going to get there. Maybe you have a plan to meet a partner, to settle down and to have a family. Maybe you want to start your own business one day and you're working on a plan to make it a reality. Maybe you want to retire early and travel the world. This is what I mean by having direction. It's a shorter-term view than your overall life purpose.

As adults we spend a lot of our time working and so having a job we enjoy and which is fulfilling is key to our everyday happiness and well-being. Work and career often fit under the medium-term direction goal.

I remember the pressure which I felt after leaving school as I didn't have a clue what I wanted to do with my life. I too had this notion that there was one vocation which I was supposed to be doing and I just hadn't worked it out yet. Thinking that there is only one job or one role for you puts a lot of pressure on you to find that one thing. You also want to find it quickly too. After all, life is short and you should be living your purpose straight away, shouldn't you?

I'll be honest; I never found this 'one job' which I should be doing from a vocation point of view. I soon learnt that life is about the journey and no one knows all the details of that journey ahead of time. You are completely in control of the roads which you take. You can set the course and direction and you are free to take a new fork in the road any time you choose to. So, in the words of my teenager, "chill out." Life is supposed to be fun!

According to the Bureau of Labor Statistics (a U.S. government agency investigating labor economics and statistics), nowadays the average person has 12 jobs in their lifetime and this number is increasing with each generation. The days of a job for life are few and far between. I have had many different roles during my journey so far from customer service representative, market researcher, marketeer, business manager, account director, project manager, full time mother, holistic therapist, author.

So, I'm here to tell you to be easy with yourself. You have choices and can change track any time if you change your mind. It is documented that around the age of 40 or 50 some people can go through a mid-life crisis. People look at their lives to date and wonder if this is all that there is. It is a good time to reflect and make changes for the next phase of life. Remember, you always have a choice.

To find meaningful, fulfilling jobs or hobbies, start by asking yourself the following questions:

- What do you love to do?

- What activities make you happy?

- What activities give you energy?

- When are you at your best? What are you doing?

- What are your key strengths?

- If money was no object, how would you spend your time?

Answers to these questions will help you to find activities and careers which you will be happy pursuing. If you don't know what gives you energy or what you love doing, then keep trying new things until you do. Ask a cross section of people you know e.g. friends, family, work colleagues or previous work colleagues, what they see as your key strengths. Sometimes, others can see strengths in us which we just can't see for ourselves.

You may find that your job or career isn't what makes you happy or energises you. However, it may pay you well and you don't have the option to change at the moment. If this is you, then look for ways to bring your passions alive in your day-to-day life. Is there anything which you could change about your current job which would make it more fulfilling? Is there a hobby or activity which you could be doing outside of work to satisfy your dreams?

Take some time now to review and to write down your direction. What are you working towards over the next few years? What would you like to achieve?

3 Goals

Goals are the shorter-term objectives which you are working towards on a monthly, weekly and daily basis. Do you have a goal which you are currently working towards?

You could have a number of shorter-term goals on a variety of subjects. For example, if you have a job then you may have been set some annual goals or objectives to achieve. But have you set yourself any personal goals? Do you have a fitness goal, a nutritional goal, a family goal or, a home goal?

These shorter-term goals help us to focus on a day-to-day basis and they give us purpose to our regular activities. I will talk more about how to set goals in section four, however having these goals helps us to stay motivated and they keep moving us forward. Once we see progress (by recording our daily wins) this also helps to build our self-esteem and encourages us to keep going and to be more positive.

You do need to have a purpose or a reason or a goal for getting out of bed each day. Once you have identified yours and you connect with it daily, then undoubtedly your spiritual wellness will improve. A purpose helps you to see how you are contributing, how you are helping and how you are adding value to the world. Once you love what you do and you are living your life on purpose, then you will feel happier and more fulfilled.

2 Spiritual / Energy Healing

Have you ever experienced spiritual/energy healing for yourself? Are you aware what it is or how it could help you?

Let's start with what exactly is spiritual/energy healing.

There are many definitions of spiritual healing. This is the current definition from the NFSH (National Federation of Spiritual Healing) Healing Trust:

> "A treatment that involves the transfer of energy through the healer to the recipient. It promotes self-healing by relaxing the body, releasing tensions and strengthening the body's own immune system. Healing is natural and non-invasive with the intention of bringing the recipient into a state of balance and well-being on all levels."

Spiritual healing is not linked to a particular faith or religion. The word spiritual comes from the Latin word that means 'breath of life.' Spiritual healing is indeed spiritual energy working at a deep level on the spiritual being. The healer is not creating the energy. The healing energy is not coming from the healer and

Spiritual Well-Being

the healer is not passing on their own energy. The role of the healer is to tune into the healing energy of the universe and then to be a vehicle through which the healing energy flows to the person receiving the healing. The healer acts as a channel connecting this Universal Energy (which helps the body, mind and spirit), to the receiving client or patient. The role of the healer is to feel, to tune in and to sense where to direct this healing energy for maximum benefit. The client or patient will receive the healing energy which he or she allows themselves to receive.

Another way to explain it is to imagine electricity, a plug and an appliance. The electricity supply is comparable to the Universal Energy, a constant supply which never runs out. It is always there but we can't necessarily see it flowing in our houses. The appliance, such as a kettle, toaster or hair dryer, is the client and the plug is the healer. In order for the appliance to receive the flow of electricity, it needs to be plugged in. The plug bridges the gap. It accesses the electricity and allows it to flow to the appliance so that it works effectively. This, in essence, is what the healer is doing during a healing session. They are the vehicle through which the Universal Energy flows to the client. It is of course possible for anyone to open themselves to receive the Universal Energy directly without a healer. They can become their own plug if you like, but that is a subject for another book.

So, what happens during a healing session? The healer tunes into the client's energy. The healer may be led to work in the aura, which is the energy that surrounds each physical body and which has many layers, or they may be led to work on the chakras (energy centres) of the body. Depending on the technique being used, the healer may place their hands on the client or they may not. In terms of effectiveness and the client's ability to receive the healing, there is no difference between hands-on and hands-off healing. It is normally down to the preference of the healer and client as to which is practised.

The human body has seven key energy centres, commonly known as chakras. Chakra is the Sanskrit word for 'wheel' or 'circle'. The chakras in the body are wheels of energy which, when whole and balanced, spin and allow energy to flow up the spine. Each chakra vibrates at a different frequency, has a unique colour and is also the energy centre for a certain area of the body. Our chakras develop over time from the moment we are born until we are 49 years old. Each chakra has a dominant focus for 7 years and has more influence over our energy during this period. Once we reach 49, the chakra cycle starts again, so the base chakra develops for another seven years and so on. Let's have a quick look at the different chakras, their functions and their influence over the human body.

Root / Base Chakra

The root chakra sits at the base of the spine and helps us to feel grounded and connected to the Earth.

Colour – Red

Development – 1 to 7 years

Sacral Chakra

The sacral chakra sits in the abdomen about two inches below the naval. It relates to the emotions and sexual energy.

Colour – Orange

Development – 8 to 14 years

Solar Plexus Chakra

The solar plexus is in the abdomen in the stomach area below the rib cage. This chakra relates to self-confidence and self-esteem.

Colour – Yellow

Development – 15 to 21 years

Heart Chakra

The heart chakra is in the middle of the chest and bridges the lower and upper chakras. This chakra controls love and inner peace.

Colour – Green

Development – 22 to 28 years

Throat Chakra

Located in the throat, this chakra allows the communication of personal power and truth.

Colour – Light blue / turquoise

Development – 29 to 35 years

Third Eye Chakra

Located in the forehead between the eyes, this chakra controls the ability to see the bigger picture and to connect to intuition.

Colour – Dark Blue / Purple

Development – 36 to 42 years

Crown Chakra

Located at the top of the head, representing the ability to truly connect spiritually to the higher self and to universal consciousness.

Colour – White

Development – 43 to 49 years.

As you can see, every seven years we have a dominant chakra which is developing. The first year of a chakra cycle is influenced by the new dominant chakra and the subsequent years are a combination of the dominant chakra and the next corresponding chakra. For example:

1st year	influenced by base chakra
2nd year	influenced by base chakra and sacral chakra
3rd year	influenced by base chakra and solar plexus chakra
4th year	influenced by base chakra and heart chakra
Etc..	

Our full chakra development takes 49 years and has many influences on us during this period. For example, during our early years, the root chakra development is our main influence and this is when, as children, we are understanding and developing our roots, where values are instilled and where we understand the meaning of home. During the years eight to fourteen our sacral chakra develops which is strongly linked to puberty and our sexual energy.

Now that I am coming to the end of my first round of chakra development it is interesting to sit back and review the different stages. I didn't know at the time, but my anxiety and panic attacks, which started in my late teens, corresponded with the development of my solar plexus chakra which is all to do with self-confidence and self-esteem. That's not to say that this is normal and will happen to anyone else, but the issues which I was facing at that point in my life also related to the emotional chakra which was developing. It took a lot of searching and understanding of events later in my life to release the negative energy which had built up and to help me overcome this programme which I had created. As I said earlier on in this section, all three well-being facets are intertwined, spiritual well-being and mental well-being influencing each other the most.

When we experience stress or negative emotions, for example fear, sadness, guilt, jealousy, anger, worry, doubt, disappointment or frustration, our chakras can become blocked. When a chakra is blocked or out of balance, neighbouring chakras compensate and these can then become overactive or underactive. This means that they are not vibrating at their normal optimum frequency. The effects of blocked chakras on the body can manifest themselves in different ways for different people. An unbalanced chakra can sometimes show up as physical ailments, emotional issues, health issues or mental blocks to name but a few examples.

By connecting a person to the Universal Healing Energy, blocks can be removed, energy restored, balance regained, and the person being healed can feel the benefits. When all of the chakras are open, clear and balanced, energy can flow freely and there is balance and peace between the body, mind and spirit.

Anyone can learn to re-balance their own chakras through meditation, self-energy healing, yoga or crystals or, if this is all new to you, you can find a qualified healer to help you. As with all therapies, I would recommend that you ask friends, family and people whom you trust for a referral and always have a 'get to know' session beforehand to make sure that you feel comfortable in the presence of the healer. It's OK if you don't feel comfortable. Not everyone has an energy which you gel with. That's why it's so important to meet first before any healing takes place. Face to face is best as it is not always easy to sense someone's energy over the internet or the telephone. Always trust your gut feeling. It will never let you down. Did you feel good whilst you were with this person? Did you come away with a good feeling or not?

Reiki

There are a number of different names for energy healing. Reiki may be a term which you have heard of or come across before. It is a specific type of energy healing originating from Japan. Reiki is predominantly hands-on-healing, where the healer attunes to the Universal Energy and this flows through the healer to the person receiving the healing. The Reiki healer will normally follow a specific sequence when giving healing and is tuned to the same Universal Energy as other energy healing methods.

Distant Healing

Distant healing is also extremely effective. As healing is conducted at an energy level, the healer doesn't necessarily need to be with the client at the time. It is possible for the healer to tune into the client and his/her energy from a distance. In these instances, it is recommended that the healer and client agree on a specific time and that both parties are in a quiet space so that the healer can tune in and the client can experience the healing albeit from afar. Not all healers offer this kind of healing but it is worth exploring if you and your healer live in different parts of the country or indeed in different countries.

Healing Benefits

Having experienced energy healing for myself and having also practiced it for many years, I am a firm believer in energy healing and the benefits which people can experience. More and more research is being conducted in the area of alternative therapies versus modern medicine and there is considerably more information online than ever before. I don't think that healing techniques should necessarily replace traditional medicine, but I do whole heartedly believe that the two can work hand in hand. Some of the benefits of energy healing which can be experienced are:

- improved harmony and balance
- reduced tension in the body
- cleared energy blocks and balanced body, mind and spirit
- clearer minds and improved focus
- peaceful mind
- improved sleep
- accelerated self-healing ability
- healed physical conditions
- an overall sense of calm and well-being.

If you've never experienced energy healing before then I would encourage you to experience the benefits for yourself. Do you personally know anyone who has regular healing? If so, ask them for a recommended practitioner. You can also search the NFSH and Reiki associations in the UK for practitioners in your local neighbourhood, or there may be a healing centre near you. In terms of results, some people receive a benefit after just one session, whilst for others it takes longer. Do what feels right for you. Relax and enjoy the experience. It's all good.

3 Hypnotherapy

Have you ever considered Hypnotherapy to help a specific area in your life?

Where Hypnotherapy Can Help

Hypnotherapy helped me through my anxiety, but this is not the only issue that it can help with. Hypnotherapy can be beneficial in numerous situations:

- helping people to stop a certain behaviour such as smoking, nail biting or drinking

- building people's confidence i.e. helping people to be able to speak in public, not to blush when spoken to, to stop stammering etc.

- solving deep rooted issues such as panic attacks, chronic pain and anxiety

- helping people to overcome phobias and fears

- solving sleep disorders such as insomnia

- Helping people to manage stress by promoting calm and relaxation.

Is there anything in your life which is currently holding you back? Is there anything which you would like to change but believe that it is deeply rooted somewhere in your subconscious?
If so, then hypnotherapy may be a good solution for you.

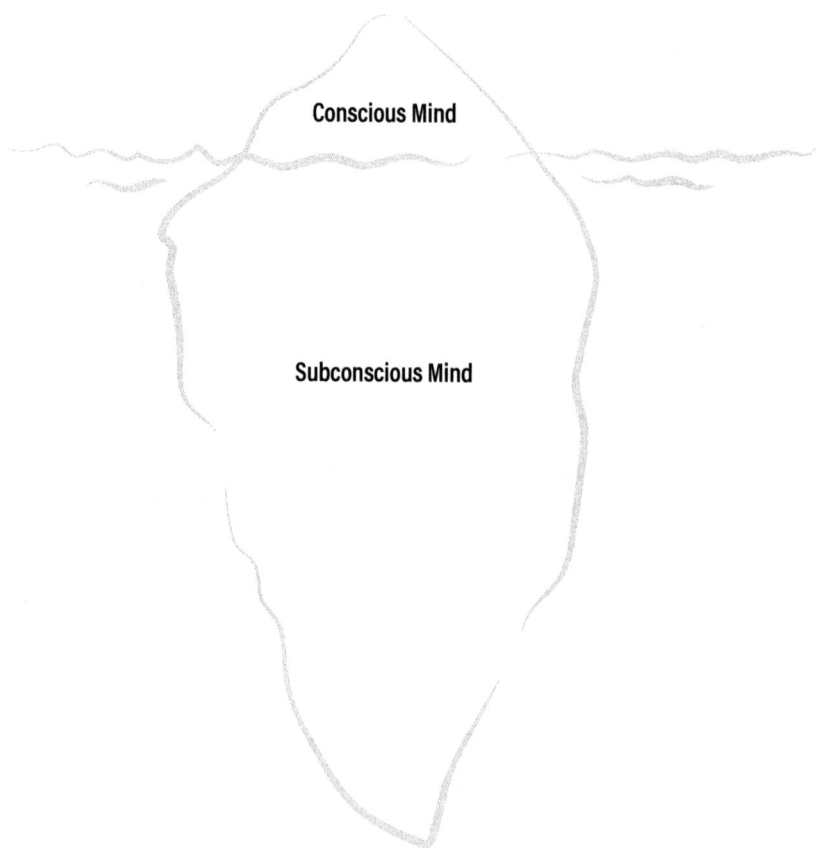

Conscious Mind

Subconscious Mind

Iceberg diagram

Let's Look At How Hypnotherapy Works

Every situation, every event and every conversation we have ever experienced, from the time we were born to where we are right now, is stored somewhere in our subconscious minds. Sit and reflect on the previous sentence just for a moment. Every single event or word spoken in your entire current physical life has been stored. How incredible is that? This amount of data is just too much to try to visualise and probably can't even be quantified but, hopefully, this paints you a picture of just how much bigger your subconscious mind is compared to your conscious mind.

It is not possible to readily remember all of these events or conversations unless they resonated with us at the time when they occurred. This is when they stay in our conscious memory. We easily have access to all memories which we have chosen to remember, which were significant for some reason. Some of these may be good and some may be bad. These conscious memories account for around 10% of our memory. 90% of our memories are stored away in this other memory bank, which is our subconscious, as illustrated in the Iceberg diagram.

We don't need to have access to the majority of our memories and events, so having this information carefully packed away in our subconscious mind is actually a good thing. We already have over 50,000 thoughts running through our conscious minds on a daily basis and we really don't need to be adding to it unnecessarily. However, sometimes it is useful to be able to recall things which have happened in the past, or access certain thoughts, beliefs and events in order for us to understand why we believe certain things, why we react in certain ways and why an issue has now surfaced at a particular point in our lives. This is where hypnotherapy comes into play. I am a strong believer that there is a reason for everything. You should access your subconscious if you want to understand why you believe what you do today, why you think like you do, why you act like you do and why you are like you are. It is this part of your mind which holds the key to your knowledge, your understanding and, ultimately, your healing.

Hypnotherapy Process

My first experience of hypnotherapy was not what I expected, probably because I had an image in my head of the hypnosis I had seen on television involving people dancing with mops and buckets or jumping around the stage pretending to be frogs. Surely, I thought, these people couldn't possibly remember what they were doing once they were de-hypnotised? I therefore expected not to remember anything of the session and I am glad to say that this was not at all the case. During my session I just felt deeply relaxed and calm. I could hear the music and I could also hear everything my therapist was saying during the hypnotherapy and, I could also remember everything afterwards too. I soon came to understand that, although a small percentage of people can go into a very deep hypnotic trance very quickly, the majority of people do not experience this at all. The process of hypnotherapy is to relax and to quieten the conscious mind in order to open up and to access the subconscious mind. It is, in essence, a very deep meditation. So, you will be fully aware of everything which is going on.

Hypnotherapy definitely helped me through a period of anxiety in my early twenties. I learnt techniques which I could put into practice whenever I felt a panic attack coming along and this in turn helped me to once again feel in control, knowing that this one would also pass if I took certain steps.

Hypnotherapy helped me to once again be able to plan events, to go on holiday and to agree to going to places which had an element of the unknown. I still worried before these events, but I didn't stop going, as I knew that I could control my breathing and get through the panic attack as and when and if it happened.

For some people, this is enough. Having some tools and techniques which they can use to calm a panic attack before it starts or, knowing coping strategies to implement when an attack is happening, is all some people need to recover. This knowledge for a lot of people helps to dispel the fear of a panic attack and can stop them from happening ever again.

However, for me, they were still happening and hindering various aspects of my life. I was also still wondering why they happened and what the reason was behind why they had started so suddenly out of nowhere. Afterall, I had gone 18 years of my life without one, so why had they started when they did? Why were they happening so frequently? And why did I feel so helpless and powerless now that they were part of my life? I questioned my hypnotherapist about this and said that I needed to understand the 'why' and not just have the 'what to do' in my armoury.

To delve deeper and to understand why, we needed to access my subconscious mind and rummage through it until we found the key events which had contributed to this new unwanted behaviour that I was experiencing. This form of hypnotherapy is known as regression therapy. Regression therapy is a powerful form of hypnotherapy and it can help to unlock past experiences or events which we have completely forgotten about. These events have been stored in the subconscious mind and, the conscious mind will not be able to identify the answers, no matter how hard we sit and think about a subject.

For regression therapy, a therapist takes their client into a very deep level of relaxation/hypnosis. The conscious mind is parked in a favourite spot, somewhere in nature for example, where it can rest, whilst the therapist continues to take the client on a journey to open up and access the subconscious mind. Only a qualified therapist should do this exercise so please do seek out a therapist who is experienced in this type of hypnotherapy. During this journey, certain questions are asked to the subconscious mind to find related events or triggers and, whilst a person is in this deep relaxation, past events and conversations can come to mind, which can be talked about and shared and in some cases re-lived from a safe vantage point.

During regression therapy it is also possible to re-train the subconscious mind, to re-write some of these events and experiences from the point of view of now being an adult or now being wiser than when the event occurred. Endings can be re-written, feelings can be changed during and after events and more beneficial thoughts and feelings around the experience can be instilled. It really is a very powerful therapy indeed.

I discovered key events which were contributing to my situation which I had no idea were related in the slightest. I had no conscious recollection of these events. My subconscious mind had packed them away whilst I was a lot younger, clearly for another day when I could understand their significance. It was truly an enlightening process and one which I was extremely grateful to experience. With the knowledge of why these panic attacks had started along with the tools and techniques which I could put into action when I felt one coming along, I once again felt back in control of my life and was able to move forward with a stronger degree of confidence.

So, if you have something in your life which is currently holding you back then hypnotherapy could be your answer.

I would encourage you to find a reputable therapist or maybe ask friends and family for a recommendation. I would also suggest that you meet with the therapist for a 'meet and greet' session before embarking on any hypnotherapy. It is beneficial to understand the process beforehand so that you feel relaxed and at ease during your first session. Having a good rapport and feeling comfortable with your hypnotherapist is also key to achieving a successful outcome.

A Quick Word On HypnoBirthing

I am very passionate about HypnoBirthing and wanted to quickly mention it here. It is a childbirth method which uses self-hypnosis techniques.

It didn't take long for the horror stories to start when I shared with friends and colleagues my news that I was expecting a baby. It seemed to be some kind of rite of passage that all existing mums felt the need to impart their birthing stories to newly pregnant ladies, in the hope of getting them prepared for the worst. It was almost like a badge of honour which women wore in terms of the length of their labours. I remember feeling truly horrified! Did these women really think that these stories were going to help me during the next few months? Would these stories help me to look forward to birthing day and enjoy my pregnancy or would they leave me with a sense of foreboding and dreading the final event? The good news however was that it made me think for myself. I always like to find an alternative so I set out to find another way.

Luckily, I remembered a unit in my hypnotherapy course which studied hypnotherapy, surgery and anesthesia. Cases were documented where patients had been able to achieve a very deep level of hypnosis which had meant that they didn't need any anesthesia for their operations. These patients were in a state of deep hypnosis during their procedures where they were able to shut off their feeling valves and they didn't feel any pain whatsoever. On researching further, I discovered HypnoBirthing for comfortable, pain-free childbirth. I was immediately sold and signed my husband and I up for our first class.

I birthed both my children using HypnoBirthing. I had no pain relief on either occasion. I was just in a very deep state of meditation. I was aware of everything which was going on around me and could communicate with my husband and midwife as needed. The births were very short, five hours and two hours respectively and I can genuinely say, hand on heart, that I felt calm and in control. I loved the feeling of being so in tune with my body and baby, that I instinctively knew what to do. Some people have questioned me over the years and commented that I must have had very small babies to be able to do this. I will let you answer that for yourself as my son was 8lb 7oz and my daughter was 9lb 13oz. I have said on more than one occasion that I would be quite happy to give birth again, anytime. For me, the parenting is the challenging part! If I had any doubt beforehand that we were all part of a spiritual world, I knew without a shadow of a doubt after birthing my children that we are part of something so much bigger than ourselves.

One of the key lessons which HypnoBirthing taught me was that we really can learn to control our minds. HypnoBirthing exercises replaced negative beliefs/images with new knowledge and positive thoughts. The meditation, which I practised daily, conditioned my mind to instantly relax when I heard this specific music. This meant that when the birthing day arrived, it would be easy for my conscious mind to be put to one side and I could let my body do what it knew to do instinctively. Also by repeating positive affirmations multiple

Simply Well-Being

times, I reprogrammed my mind that birthing would be a comfortable, pain-free experience.

I went into both my births believing that they would be pain-free, that my mind and body would relax and that my body would instinctively know what to do. I was able to re-condition and manage my mind and my thoughts and take control. As a result, I know without a shadow of a doubt that we can be in complete control of our minds and bodies; they need not be in control of us.

So, for any young people reading this book, or indeed pregnant ladies or couples, I would encourage you to look into HypnoBirthing as an option for delivering your newborn into this world. The tools and techniques not only help you through your pregnancy journey and birthing but also into parenthood as well. My birthing stories are so very different to most other women and I want to be a beacon of hope that birthing can actually be a very enjoyable experience. **www.hypnobirthing. org**

4 Spiritual Response Therapy (SRT)

Spiritual Response Therapy (SRT) is not as well-known as some other therapies, but it is a very powerful and effective healing therapy which I wanted to share with you.

My dad introduced me to it a year or so after my son was born. I was itching to learn something new and to get my mind working again so I did some research and then signed myself up. It sounded fascinating and I was eager to know more. It also felt like it was the next logical step after hypnotherapy in terms of releasing negative energy and blocks quickly and effectively.

The course took place over a three-day weekend and I completed it with five other people including my mum and dad. It was very intense as there was a lot to learn, but we also spent a lot of time clearing ourselves of negative energy and blocks which we had gained. I can honestly say that when I arrived home, I felt so much lighter as though pressure had been released from my head and shoulders. The benefit is difficult to put into words, but on arriving back into the office on the Monday morning, two colleagues commented on how different I looked. Had I done something different with my hair? Did I have new glasses? Was I wearing my make up differently? The answer to all of those questions was, "No." There was nothing tangibly or visibly different about me, but inside I did feel free and I was walking a little bit taller, so maybe that is what these two colleagues could sense.

So, What Is Spiritual Response Therapy (SRT)?

SRT is a quick and very effective, painless healing technique which releases blocks and negative energy from our energy space. It is a system of researching the subconscious mind and Akashic records to quickly find the blocks, the limitations and the negativity which is being held onto. These are then released and replaced with loving energy, supportive ideas and positive beliefs.

Akashic records, according to the religion of theosophy and the philosophical school called anthroposophy, are a comprehensive collection of all universal events, thoughts, words, emotions and intent ever to have occurred in the past, present or future, in terms of all entities and life forms, not just human. (Wikipedia definition)

The philosophy is that everyone has a set of Akashic records which hold that person's entire history, including everything which has ever happened to that spirit or soul in this life and in all of its past lives, parallel lives and future lives. Everything is stored here in the Akashic records and you have full access to any information about your history and Akashic records via your higher self.

Your higher self is your spiritual self as opposed to your physical self. Every one of us has a higher self. This is part of who we are spiritually. Some say it is our true selves and some say it is our inner guidance system. Our higher self is the part of us which is linked to the spirit world and connected to the Universal Energy. Our higher self is an extension of who we are, it is not a separate entity. It is what speaks to us when we meditate, when we dream and when we imagine. It is our inner knowing and our wise counsel.

In the hypnotherapy chapter, I explained that our subconscious minds hold every memory from this life we are living right now on earth. We can also access past lives from our subconscious minds as well. Our Akashic records hold further knowledge of every experience, every event and every emotion from all of our lives and from all dimensions, past, present and future.

SRT is non-denominational. Your religion does not matter. It can help anyone and everyone as it is a spiritual healing method. However, it does work on the belief that souls have incarnated before and that they will incarnate again. It looks at past lives, present lives and future lives. SRT also demonstrates that our souls tend to reincarnate with other soul family members time and time again. Every re-incarnation can be a different sex, a different role in a family or a different generation.

This might be a new concept to some of you, so let me give you some examples. Have you ever had a feeling when you meet someone for the first time that you've met them before or that you feel like you know them, even though you've never met in this lifetime? Have you ever met someone and immediately hit it off, felt comfortable in their presence and felt like you have known this person for years? When this happens, it is your soul recognising their soul. You have probably met many times before in previous lives and your souls are remembering the past lives which you have lived together. When this happens, it's not uncommon for one person to acknowledge that they feel like they know this person and the other person agrees as they feel the same. This has happened to me many times during my life and each time it makes me smile, as I know my path has crossed with this person in a different lifetime.

SRT works on the premise that we get to choose to reincarnate back into the physical world. We choose to take on new roles, new circumstances and new genders. For example, your spouse in this life may or may not have been your spouse in a previous life. Maybe he or she was a parent or a sibling or a close friend. Stories and situations can easily be researched using SRT. It really is fascinating when you get started.

So, How Can Spiritual Response Therapy (SRT) Help You With Your Well-Being?

It is probable that you have carried through negative events, blocks and patterns into this present life and these can manifest at any time during your current life. Maybe you have a pattern of behaviour in this life which is limiting you. Maybe you keep making the same mistakes over and over again. Maybe you have conflict which you would like to resolve or a phobia which has manifested from nowhere. All these situations could be linked to events which happened a long time ago. SRT can be used to identify all the related events quickly, pinpointing the negative energy which you continue to carry today. SRT can then release the negative energy which is not serving you anymore and replace it with love and universal healing energy. Once released and replaced with positive energy, patterns are broken, emotions disappear, phobias and anxiety can subside and blocks are released so that you, the client, can then move forward with your life.

Think of your Akashic records as a massive story book entitled 'You.' Everything about you from the beginning of time is stored in this book. Your higher self has access to these records and can quickly and easily find the right information that you are looking for once the right questions are asked. Sit for a moment and re-read the last three sentences. What a fascinating book your Akashic records is. What would you like to know? What would you like to ask?

Simply Well-Being

Where Spiritual Response Therapy (SRT) Can Help

SRT is effective in so many ways and can really help people to flourish in this life and beyond. SRT is effective in helping:

- clearing anxiety and unwanted behaviours and phobias
- clearing blocks on money, love, happiness, romantic engagements and clearing family tensions
- releasing repeated behavioural patterns and breaking habits
- helping make life decisions (the practitioner can identify the percentage of negative and positive energy towards your questions and decisions).

What happens during an SRT session?

To begin a session, the SRT practitioner carries out a 'preparation to work' where the practitioner's higher self links with the client's higher self. Once the SRT practitioner's higher self is speaking to the client's higher self, then the practitioner can start the clearing process. This entails asking specific questions, depending on what the client is hoping to achieve, and the answers are shown via a pendulum and specific charts. SRT uses muscle responses to bypass the conscious mind to connect with the subconscious mind and soul records.

The practitioner can quickly identify the root causes of any discordant/negative energy or issues. The discordant/negative energy is then released and replaced with positive loving energy leaving a new positive life experience.

The practitioner will talk the client through everything which they are doing and finding as they go through the clearing process. Alternatively, a practitioner may choose to complete the session and then explain the findings and healings at the end, either verbally or as a written summary.

There are two main approaches to SRT:

1. Researching a specific issue which the client may be experiencing.

2. Conducting a full clearing session. This option will bring to light the main issues and discordant energy which is affecting the client in the here and now, as well as situations which the client is not even aware of which could be affecting or influencing them.

The practitioner will identify those negative energies, programs (repeated behaviours), soul contracts (a promise which you made before reincarnating which is now holding you back) and blocks which are inhibiting you from leading a happy, healthy and fulfilled life in the here and now. The practitioner will communicate what stories are being explained, what events are being shown and what negative energies are being released. It really is a fascinating process to watch come together.

SRT Benefits

A huge benefit of SRT versus hypnotherapy is the speed at which the therapist can uncover certain events and situations which are causing issues for clients. As discussed earlier, hypnotherapy can use regression therapy to take a person back in time to discover root causes. Although extremely effective, in some instances these events or past experiences can be very painful and emotional to re-live again. With SRT, the higher self identifies the event and the related emotions and negative energy which is being held by the client by asking specific questions. It is then relatively painless, quick and easy to release this negative energy without the client having to personally re-live the event.

During SRT it is possible to identify scenarios from past lives, identifying when, what and who was involved and then correlating them to the people who are in your life currently. It is honestly a fascinating subject when you start to explore it. You learn to understand why you act certain ways with various people and why you are feeling the way you do towards them. It may have absolutely nothing to do with what they recently said or have done to you. It may well run deeper to a different lifetime and you are just re-living the same negative energy in the here and now.

Do you have any issues or problems which you just haven't been able to solve by any other means? Do you have any phobias or irrational fears which have recently surfaced in your life for no reason? Are you feeling stuck and want to move forward feeling positive and happy?

If you have answered yes to any of these questions, then SRT may well be a solution for you. To find out more on this fascinating therapy or, if you would like to find a practitioner in your area to speak to then I would encourage you to visit the SRT website which is: www.spiritualresponse.com

I also recommend the book by Robert E Detzler – The Freedom Path.

5 Hands-on Healing Therapies

Hands-on healing therapies could very well sit within the physical well-being section of this book. However, I believe that they are best placed here in the spiritual section as they not only have a positive effect on our physical bodies but on our spiritual well-being as well.

Indian Head Massage

Have you experienced the benefits of an Indian Head Massage?

Do you sit hunched over a laptop all day? Do you experience frequent neck and shoulder pain from stress? Do you struggle to relax? Do you suffer with frequent headaches or migraines? If you have answered yes to any of these questions, then this therapy could be your solution.

Indian head massage is a treatment which focuses on massaging acupressure points along the shoulders, neck and head. It is derived from Ayurvedic traditions (Ayurvedic is a natural system of medicine, originating in India 3,000 years ago) and uses a variety of massage techniques to release negative blockages of energy. It is a very gentle therapy, extremely relaxing and has a multitude of both physiological and psychological benefits. The benefits can include:

- deep relaxation, reducing stress and anxiety

- relief from mental fatigue and clearer thought and concentration

- increased blood flow to the shoulders, neck and head thus stimulating hair follicles and encouraging skin cell regeneration

- easing and prevention of migraines, headaches, neck and shoulder pain

- soothing the sinuses and aiding decongestion

- energising and helping to renew and balance energy levels

- relief of muscular tension

- improvement of mood.

The treatment can be delivered seated or in a specific massage therapy chair. The therapist starts the treatment from the top of the back and shoulders before moving on to the neck, head and face. The treatment normally lasts around 30 minutes. Before a treatment, the therapist should conduct a consultation to ascertain the suitability of the treatment for you, the client, and to answer any questions which you may have.

After the treatment you will be encouraged to drink plenty of water, as toxins will have been released during the treatment and drinking water helps to prevent any headaches as a result. You should feel relaxed with less tension after the treatment.

One of the benefits of Indian head massage is that it can be carried out without having to remove any clothing and as such is a simple and effective treatment to be carried out at the workplace. At one of my forward-thinking corporate companies, we had a therapist who would be on-site during lunchtimes and you could book a 20 minute head massage.

Simply Well-Being

The benefits could clearly be seen amongst employees. They were less stressed, calmer and happier in their work.

Massage

Do you spend the majority of your day seated in a chair? Do you experience shoulder or back pain? Do you suffer with stress or anxiety? Do you have trouble sleeping or relaxing? Do you have any repetitive strain injuries? Do you suffer with headaches or migraines? Massage can help if you answered yes to any of these questions.

The history of massage therapy dates back to 3,000 BC (or earlier) in India where it was considered a sacred system of natural healing. Used by Hindus in Ayurvedic medicine (alternative natural medicine), massage therapy was a practise passed down through generations to help heal injuries, relieve pain and to prevent and cure illnesses.

There are many different forms and types of massage these days. Finding a therapist who is right for you will ensure you have the best experience. I have experienced many massages over the years, some significantly better than others. Yes, it is worth asking around for a recommendation but, if you don't receive the type of massage you were hoping for, then move on to the next therapist. Everyone has their own personal preference in terms of pressure applied, oils or no oils, full body or just back, neck and shoulders. To gain the most benefit you need to find a therapist who suits your needs.

There are many different types of massage, including Swedish, Thai, shiatsu, hot stone, aromatherapy, deep tissue, sports and pre-natal. There are many books on the various different techniques however here is a quick overview of the differences:

Swedish – also known as the 'traditional' massage. The therapist uses oil and applies the main massage techniques to the areas being treated.

Thai – works the entire body and is one of the most invigorating massages as the therapist moves the body into yoga stretches.

Shiatsu – integrates emotional, psychological and spiritual well-being. It combines finger pressure on different pressure points, gentle stretches and, in some cases, meditation.

Hot stone – the therapist places hot stones along the spine and then uses the stones to massage the back. The heat is a great way to relax muscles and increase overall relaxation.

Aromatherapy – the therapist uses a specific blend of aromatherapy oils during the massage based on the needs of the client.

Deep tissue – focuses on relieving severe muscle tension. The therapist will work deeply using thumbs, knuckles and elbows to really get to the problem areas.

Pre-natal – specifically for pregnant women. Only specific oils should be used during pregnancy so finding a qualified pre-natal massage therapist is important. As lying on the stomach is not possible after the first trimester, pre-natal massage uses different positions to accommodate the client's shape.

A massage therapist will perform various massage strokes that warm and work muscle tissue, releasing tension and breaking up muscle knots or adhered tissues, called adhesions. This in turn promotes relaxation, eases muscle tension, and creates other health benefits.

Lactic acid, metabolic by-products and waste that build up over time can be removed through the use of massage therapy treatments. When treating injured muscles, massage helps decrease tension and release toxins through the use of stretching and manual techniques. There are four main massage techniques which are incorporated into a massage session:

Effleurage – light or deep stroking. This is meant for relaxation and the release of tension.

Petrisage – kneading, which helps to relieve muscle spasms.

Tapotement – tapping or chopping, which helps to break down knots.

Friction – small circular motions and concentration of pressure on a particular point, which releases tension in specific spots.

Massage Benefits

Not only can massage produce physical benefits but it can also produce strong emotional benefits too. Massage triggers an involuntary, but welcome, relaxation response from the nervous system. This causes the heart and breathing rates to slow down and the blood pressure and stress hormones to decrease. This counteracts the negative effects of emotional stress. The benefits of massage are extensive and include:

- relief of stress
- reduction of anxiety

- relief of postoperative pain

- management of low-back pain

- reduction of muscle tension

- relief of tension headaches

- overall feeling of caring for yourself

- feeling of well-being and calm.

Treatments can last between 30 and 90 minutes depending on the type of massage which you have booked. At the end of a treatment, it is recommended to drink plenty of water. The water helps to flush the toxins, which have been released during the massage, out of your system. If they are not flushed out, the toxins hang around in the blood stream and kidneys and, as a result, people can sometimes experience a headache after the treatment.

Massage is a wonderful complementary therapy to aid traditional medicine, especially for emotional illnesses such as anxiety and stress. Your therapist may recommend a series of treatments or you may benefit from just the one. Everyone is individual and unique.

Reflexology

Reflexology is one of my favourite hands-on healing treatments to receive myself. It treats the whole body even though the therapy focuses on hands and feet.

Reflexology is the application of pressure or massage to specific points on the feet or hands. Modern reflexology is based on an ancient Chinese form of the therapy which has been practiced for thousands of years. It is based on the theory that various points on the feet correspond to various organs in the body and, by applying pressure to specific areas, energy blockages can be released and as a result, the body can experience relaxation and healing.

Whereas massage works on the whole body, reflexology is focused solely on the feet and the hands, working specific pressure points. Reflexologists use maps of these points on the feet and hands to determine where they should apply pressure.

The souls of the feet and hands contain thousands of nerve endings. By applying pressure to certain points, reflexology stimulates the body into healing itself by removing blockages and improving circulation.

A treatment normally lasts 45 to 60 minutes. During that time, the reflexologist will work on both feet and pay particular attention to any blockages which he or she may feel. When reflex points are blocked or congested, they may feel painful or tender when the reflexologist is working on them. However, over time the tenderness should decrease with pressure. Reflexology should not be a painful experience so let your therapist know if you experience pain or discomfort.

If you have specific issues, it is worth discussing these before the session so that your therapist can tailor the treatment accordingly and spend extra time on particular points. For example, if you explain you suffer with premenstrual syndrome (PMS) the reflexologist may well focus on your big toe and ankle to calm your reproductive system.

Like massage, there are many documented benefits of reflexology:

- boosts immune system

- improves mood and general well-being

- reduces stress and anxiety

- clears colds, bacterial infections and sinus issues
- aids recovery from back problems
- corrects hormonal imbalances
- boosts fertility
- improves digestion
- eases arthritis pain.

There are not too many research studies into reflexology, but it is widely seen as a complementary therapy to help reduce symptoms, pain and improve someone's quality of life. It should not be used to replace traditional medicine. It is a safe therapy to try and, as with all therapies, your reflexologist should carry out a consultation before any treatment to understand any pre-existing conditions and where the therapy can be most beneficial for you. A series of treatments may be necessary to help with certain ailments or just one session may suffice. The therapy works on an individual basis.

I, for one, find reflexology extremely relaxing and can feel the benefits on my overall energy after a treatment. If, however, you don't like people touching your feet, then maybe this isn't the therapy for you. But for anyone else curious to try it I would thoroughly recommend a general well-being session.

Spiritual Well-Being Next Steps

Take a minute to reflect on what you have read in this section.

Review the score which you gave your spiritual well-being at the beginning of the book. What was it? Where do you want it to be?

Which one or two topics resonated with you the most whilst you were reading this spiritual well-being section? Write them down.

What do you need to do to help your spiritual well-being to improve?

SECTION FOUR

Getting Started

Daily Well-Being Practise

I do hope that you have found some useful chapters in this book which will help you to boost and improve your daily well-being. Maybe I have introduced you to some new practises which you hadn't thought of (see Appendix two for summary) or, new therapies which you would like to try. However, if you are feeling slightly overwhelmed by all of the information and don't know where to start, then my recommendation would be to look at which area of your well-being had the lowest score when you completed the initial exercise. Then, choose one or two activities from that well-being section which have specifically resonated with you whilst reading this book. I would encourage you to write them down and then start to implement these activities on a daily basis. In order to make a long-term change or to ensure that the new activity becomes a regular habit, it is important to set some goals. Writing them down and declaring them to someone else who can hold you accountable is also good practise. Here are a few words on goal setting.

1 Goal Setting

In between Christmas and New Year, I like to take some time to reflect on the past year and to decide my new goals for the one ahead. For me, this is just good practise.

I've always been lucky enough never to have to work in between Christmas and New Year so, after the big day, I will grab a few hours to sit down and reflect on the year which was. I'll look at the goals which I set at the beginning of the year as well as my monthly goals. I'll review and write down all of the things which I have achieved and accomplished. It's a good practise to be able to identify what I could have done better and what I am proud of during the year. Of course, you don't need to wait to do this reflection once a year, you can set monthly or weekly goals and review your progress after these frequencies too.

These are some of the reflective questions which I like to ask:

- What have I achieved in my work?

- What places have I visited / holidays I have taken?

- What has been my proudest moment(s)?

- What has changed for me this year for the better?

- How have my mental, physical and spiritual well-being been throughout the year?

- What have I learnt this year? Is there anything which I would do differently next time?

- What would I like to have more of next year?

I will then start to think about the new year and what I want to achieve in the next 12 months. So, questions I will ask myself are:

- Where do I want to be this time next year / in 5 years' time?

- Where do I want to be living?

- How do I want to be spending my time?

- What are my health, fitness and well-being goals?

- What are my financial goals?

- What hobby have I always wanted to start?

- What do I want more of?

Life is always changing; that is the one thing which is guaranteed in life. Change is constant and things never stay the same. The majority of people overestimate what they can achieve in a day or week, but vastly underestimate what they can achieve in a year or longer. The reason behind this under-estimation is because our minds struggle to understand and comprehend longer periods of time. We set ourselves ridiculously long weekly 'to do' lists because a week is a period of time which our mind can identify with. We know that each week has the same seven days with the same 24 hours in each day and so it is easier for our minds to work out what it believes is achievable in this time frame. However, when we think about the period of a year, trying to allocate activities to 365 days is just too much for our minds to compute and so we end up under-calling what we can actually accomplish.

So, what does all this mean? If we are looking to be as effective as we can be and to achieve everything we set out to, we need to have different levels of goals. This means identifying

Simply Well-Being

big, overall goals (or life goals) and then identifying smaller goals or milestones which are helping us towards them.

Writing down your life and annual goals is a very interesting exercise. It not only gives you a clear direction, it also helps you to say no to all of those activities which you've been doing which aren't serving you or helping you to achieve any of your goals. When I completed this exercise, it helped me not only to prioritise my time, but I quickly became aware of all of those activities which I was doing which were not related to any of my goals. This gave me the clarity to stop certain roles which I was playing and made it easy to say yes or no to new things.

Do you ever feel like you are busy all of the time, running from one thing to the next, but you never achieve what you really want to? If you do this goal setting exercise, what you might find is that some of your 'doing activities' have nothing to do with any of your personal goals. You could find that you are spending a lot of your time helping others with their goals and not moving yours forward at the same time. This is extremely common.

Once you are clear on your goals and what you are trying to accomplish, if a new opportunity arises which doesn't fit with one of your goals, then it is easier to say no straight away. By having clarity on your goals and purpose you will find that you don't get pulled off-course so easily and you don't get sidetracked.

GOAL MAP

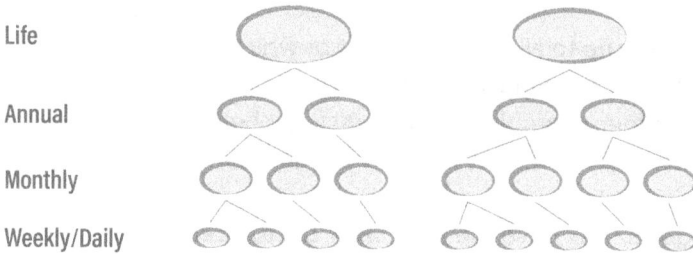

Life			
Annual			
Monthly			
Weekly/Daily			

NB: number of goals and sub goals is indicative only. Every individual goal plan will look different.

Most people have one or two life goals. These are meaty goals such as to be happy, to be successful, to leave a legacy or to make a difference. Underneath each of these life goals are annual goals or five-yearly goals which will help to achieve one of the overall life goals. Underneath the annual goal will be monthly goals and then daily or weekly tasks which need completing in order to achieve the annual goal.

Let's focus on an annual goal and look at how we can break it down. What is the one goal you would love to accomplish this year or in the next 12 months? Write it down and then spend some time chunking it down into the specific activities which you need to complete in order to make the overall goal happen. Then break these activities down even further. Are there sub-activities? How long do you think these will take you to accomplish? Knowing this will help you to build your monthly, weekly and daily goal plans. This process helps you to avoid over or underestimating what you can achieve and when.

Let's say that you have an annual goal of losing a stone in

weight. Maybe you chunk the goal down and give yourself a monthly target of how much weight you would like to lose. Maybe you set yourself an exercise goal each month in terms of activities which you are going to do and how frequently you plan to achieve them. For your weekly/daily tasks, maybe here you add how you are planning to manage your food e.g. are you following the balanced diet option? Are you following the daily calorie allowance? Are you eating whole, unprocessed food and cooking from scratch? How many meat meals are you eating? How many vegetarian meals are you eating? How much water are you drinking? Hopefully, this gives you an idea of how to set an annual goal and then how to chunk it down to the daily tasks which you need to focus on.

Writing down goals and devising a detailed action plan is critical if you are serious about achieving your objectives. Because otherwise, without a plan, a goal is just a glorified wish. Let me say that again … **a goal without a plan is just a glorified wish**.

Writing down goals on paper in your own handwriting is exceptionally powerful. Our brain uses all of our five senses when deciding whether something is true for us or not. Therefore, when it comes to our goals, we need to think them, write them down so that we can see them written in our own handwriting and we need to say the goals out loud as well, so that our brain can hear the goals too. By doing all of these things, as well as visualising the goal materialising, we are helping to cement the intention into our brain by working with the law of attraction.

Once written, goals need to be SMART: Specific, Measurable, Achievable, Realistic and Time-bound.

I've talked about making goals specific by writing them down and allocating a time frame to them. They also need to be achievable and realistic otherwise it is human nature to give up at the first hurdle.

Let's explore 'getting healthy'. Maybe you set yourself a goal of becoming a vegetarian but the reality is that you love meat, eat it every day and your hangover cure is definitely a bacon sandwich. You may do well on your first and second days, planning out some alternatives to eat and filling your fridge with fruit and vegetables. However, after a few days, you get invited out to dinner, your flat-mate starts frying bacon, your mum invites you round for a delicious Sunday roast dinner and so you cave in. You eat a meat meal and then beat yourself up that the goal was a ridiculously hard one to begin with.

Firstly, this may not be you. I do know people who have gone cold turkey literally and switched from carnivore to vegetarian overnight. It is possible, but it is not necessarily the norm. Secondly, when making a change to your way of living, it is advisable to declare it to your nearest and dearest. This not only keeps you accountable for the change but also allows them to support your new choices. And thirdly, just because you ate meat during the first week, does not mean that you should give up entirely on your goal. It might mean that you want to amend the goal slightly to allow yourself to eat meat maybe once a week until you find enough vegetarian alternatives. Or you may recognise that giving up meat completely is a step too far but increasing the number of vegetarian meals you eat in a week is completely achievable.

Starting with a goal which is achievable and realistic is important if you are to stick to it and ultimately achieve your goal.

Goals also need to be measurable. This allows you to monitor whether or not you are achieving the goal. So, whether you have a weight loss goal, a goal for the number of vegetarian meals you will eat each week, a meditation goal, a walking goal or a drinking water goal, make sure that it is measurable

Simply Well-Being

so that you can track and see progress and celebrate your success. When you can see your progress, your daily wins and your successes, this is what keeps you completing the daily action and moving forward.

So, with all of the above in mind, what are your goals for your mental, physical and spiritual well-being? Where do you want to improve? Go back to the scores out of ten which you gave each area at the beginning of the book. Where do you need to make improvements? What changes are you going to make?

Current mental well-being score out of ten

What score out of ten do I want it to be?

What is my goal?

Current physical well-being score out of ten

What score out of ten do I want it to be?

What is my goal?

Current spiritual well-being score out of ten

What score out of ten do I want it to be?

What is my goal?

2 Small, Consistent Actions

I believe the key to success for all things in life is little actions, repeated consistently. So often, when we decide to make a change in our life, we set ourselves a ridiculously challenging goal, or we decide to radically change a number of things at the same time.

Two days into the new regime we realise that we haven't seen any benefits whatsoever. Perhaps we think that the goals are too difficult to maintain, we're missing our old ways, or it's just too difficult and so we stop, give up and think that the exercise of trying to change or implement something better was a complete waste of time!

A classic example of this is when we make New Year resolutions. Many people set huge resolutions such as to stop smoking, to stop drinking, to get fit, to go to the gym every day or to lose a significant amount of weight. They go all-out at the gym on day one and two only to ache all over in places they didn't know they had. This then prevents them from going on day three and four and, before they know it, the momentum has disappeared and the only thing going to the gym regularly is the standing order which they keep meaning to cancel!

Another example is the person committed to losing a few stone who cuts out all of their favourite food on the first day, eats like a rabbit for a few days, is hungry, tired, experiences a headache, has not seen any great weight loss in the first week and very soon falls off the wagon and goes back to eating as they did before.

Can you relate to this? Have you ever set yourself a goal which was just too unrealistic without a manageable plan?

Making small, manageable, realistic changes has been proven to be a lot more effective in terms of changing bad habits into better habits. By setting realistic daily and weekly activities and committing to them, you are far more likely to continue doing them and to succeed in seeing change over time.

As a society we are being conditioned to expect instant gratification in all things. Everything should happen now and results should be quickly visible. Technology has provided information at our fingertips. We can download films, music, apps and books at record speed. We can order groceries, clothes and pretty much any item and get it delivered to our door in under 24 hours. Unfortunately though, instant gratification is not possible in every area of our lives and in reality, most things which are worthwhile having still take time.

To change your habits and lifestyle it takes time, commitment and daily practise. You need to be willing to give up ways which don't serve you to make way for good practises. These are the steps you need to go through to make some new healthy well-being habits:

1. Choose an area which you want to change.

2. Decide on the activities which will help you to improve.

3. Plan how you are going to incorporate these new tasks into your everyday life.

4. Commit to completing them daily for a period of time. Practise, practise and practise them until they become a new habit, a new normal and just something which you automatically do as part of your daily routine.

The key to making any successful change is in what you choose to do repeatedly every day. Doing something little and often and being consistent every day is the way to make positive and lasting changes.

Think about all of those skills which you have learnt over the years. Think back to your childhood. How did you learn to read? Did you plug your brain into a computer one day and the next day you could read perfectly? Of course not! You learnt by learning letters, reading words, lines and books every day for a good few years before you became a proficient reader.

When you learnt to swim, did your parents throw you into the swimming pool one day and you proceeded to swim front crawl for 30 lengths? I very much doubt it! You would have had daily or weekly swimming lessons where you built up your skills over time until they became subconscious actions.

When you watch the Olympic Games on television, have those competitors applied for a place and just turned up with the hope of being the best on the day with no training? No, they will have committed to a rigorous training programme. Then, they will have put in hours of daily training sessions consistently for months and years beforehand, to make sure that they are ready and able to compete at their best during the championships.

Every skill which you have learnt in your life has been the result of consistent daily or weekly practice to get better and better and better. Changing your well-being habits is no different.

Experts say that it takes 30 days to change your behaviour,

so I encourage you to commit to and track your progress for 30 days. Having a physical tracker, whether on paper or on your computer or phone, which you complete and look at each day will keep you accountable for the tasks which you have agreed to do.

Sometimes, when we are making a change and implementing new activities, we can have a day when we forget or when we don't complete the activity for one reason or another. Missing one day does not mean that you have failed and is not a reason to completely stop or to give up. If this happens to you, first of all ask yourself why you didn't do the activity. Secondly, refer back to your goal and why you are trying to achieve that goal. Then, make a plan as to what you will do differently next time to make sure you don't miss it again. Start with a clean slate the following day.

In essence, success depends on the Compound Effect, a strategy developed by Darren Hardy. It describes the exercise of small daily actions which, when completed daily and consistently over time, compound to deliver a much larger goal.

How many of you could get up tomorrow and run a marathon? I am one for sure who would not be able to achieve this. I may be able to run to the end of the road without keeling over, but that would probably be my limit. However, if I committed to running a marathon in 12 months' time, if I consulted a running expert, worked out a daily training plan for a little bit of running / jogging each day, over time my stamina would build. I would be able to run further and further each week until reaching my goal of being able to run a marathon in a year's time. Small doses of running or training completed daily and consistently would compound over time to ensure that I could run further than I could when I started on day one.

So, please bear the Compound Effect in mind when starting on your new daily well-being journey. It is not realistic to expect to feel radically different after seven days of activity, though you may well feel happier and mentally more positive that you have started this journey. Please remember that it is the consistent completion of these daily actions which will compound over time to help you feel well and more in control. All of your new habits will serve you extremely well in the long run.

So, now I would like you to add to your previous goals the specific activity which you are going to introduce and complete daily to help you achieve your goals.

Current mental well-being score out of ten

What score out of ten do I want it to be?

What is my goal?

What daily activity am I going to introduce to help me?

Current physical well-being score out of ten

What score out of ten do I want it to be?

What is my goal?

What daily activity am I going to introduce to help me?

Current spiritual well-being score out of ten

What score out of ten do I want it to be?

What is my goal?

What activity am I going to introduce to help me?

3 What change are you committing to?

Hopefully by now you should have your list of goals and activities which you are going to implement in order to improve your daily well-being.

You may have chosen one new activity for your mental health, one for your physical health and one for your spiritual health. For example, you might decide to meditate for 15 minutes a day, drink 1.5 litres of water and have a reflexology session once a fortnight.

Or you may have chosen to focus on just one change and to make sure that you have embedded it into your daily routine before incorporating another activity. This is an excellent start.

Whatever you have chosen, it is important to review how you are progressing. To do this, write a list of aspects related to your new activity which you hope will improve as a result. Review how you are feeling after a week, after two weeks and again after 30 days. For example, if your daily activity is to drink 1.5 litres of water every day for 30 days, the list of aspects could be:

- How is your clarity of thinking?

- How are you sleeping?

- What is your energy level?

- What is the quality of your skin?

By tracking your progress you will begin to see and feel the benefits for yourself. Having this evidence of improvement will motivate you to continue with this new action until it becomes a healthy new habit. You are also more likely to implement another change and another change and another.

Over time I have devised a series of daily well-being activities which works for me:

- 15 minutes or more movement

- good nutrition and gut health

- drink 1.5 litres of water

- meditate/quiet time 15 minutes a day

- record daily gratitude and wins

- healing session (at least once a month).

Remember that Rome was not built in a day. For any new daily action set yourself a goal for 14 days, for 30 days, for 60 days and then review after that period of time. Be kind to yourself. Any change in daily routine takes discipline and takes time. If you fail to complete on one day, do not stop. Just acknowledge why you didn't complete it. Understand what you could do in the future to stop yourself from missing it again and then re-start in the morning. That's the beauty of a new day, you can start anew. You don't need to wait until New Year's Day or the first of the month or a Monday morning. You can choose to start a new habit or to make a change any day of the week, month or year. It's entirely up to you. You just need to decide and then commit to completing the new task daily for a set period of time.

TRACKER EXAMPLE

Well-Being Activity	Mon	Tue	Wed	Thu	Fri	Sat	Sun	Mon	Tue	Wed	Thu	Fri	Sat	Sun
Drink 1.5 litres water														
10 minutes meditation														

In Summary

My goal at the beginning of this book was to provide some help, so that people can improve their daily well-being. I wanted to share my gathered knowledge on all aspects of well-being and to consider that all three areas of mental, physical and spiritual well-being are equally as important. I do hope that you have managed to find something which is useful and which you can take forward and put into daily practice. I hope I have shown you that you are in control of your own well-being and your body, mind and soul. If you know some tools and techniques which you can implement daily, as well as having a few up your sleeve for those trying times, then you will be more able to experience true well-being on your life journey.

The older I get, the more I appreciate my health and understand its importance. Our health truly is our wealth. Sit and think about that for a minute. The majority of people only seem to appreciate their health when they feel unwell or sick in some way. It is only then that their health, or lack of it at the time, is at the forefront of their minds. People then focus and spend their time wishing that they were better and in full health. We only have one physical body which we are inhabiting whilst we live in this lifetime, so prioritising it and looking after it makes sense. Remember that no one ever regretted eating healthily, no one regretted drinking a glass of water, no one regretted meditating, and no one regretted completing that workout. So how important is your well-being to you? What are you going to do differently as of tomorrow?

Don't procrastinate. Don't close this book without deciding what change you are going to make. Write it down. Declare it to your nearest and dearest. Get started.

Well-being is a continual journey, there is no end destination. I am still learning and making changes as and when necessary.

It is all about the journey.

I do hope that I have inspired you in some way to look after your well-being. I wish for you daily well-being and a continued happy, abundant life.

For more information please visit **www.simply-well-being. com**.

		Which aspect of your well-being will benefit?		
		Spiritual	Mental	Physical
Spiritual Well-Being Strategies	Finding a Purpose	yes	yes	
	Spiritual Healing	yes	yes	yes
	Hypnotherapy	yes	yes	yes
	Spiritual Response Therapy (SRT)	yes	yes	yes
	Hands-on Healing Therapies	yes	yes	yes
Mental Well-Being Strategies	Quiet time	yes	yes	
	Meditation	yes	yes	yes
	Inner Peace/nature	yes	yes	yes
	Positive self-talk		yes	
	Positive Affirmations		yes	yes
	Attitude of Gratitude		yes	
	Daily Wins		yes	
	Friends and Family		yes	
	Calm Thinking		yes	
Physical Well-Being Strategies	Nutrition		yes	yes
	Hydration		yes	yes
	Gut Health		yes	yes
	Skin Products			yes
	Exercise		yes	yes
	Rest	yes	yes	yes

Simply Well-Being

Appendix One

The strategies discussed in this book are not necessarily specific to improving just one area of our well-being. The table shows the overlap and which facets of our well-being benefits from the specific strategies.

MENTAL WELL-BEING STRATEGIES

	Try This Exercise	Suggested Action
Quiet time	5 minutes of quiet time. Breathe in to the count of four and out to the count of four.	Schedule 5 minutes of quiet time each day.
Meditation	1 Bring your attention to the here and now. Notice your five senses. What is happening right now? This is Mindfulness. 2 Close your eyes and say out loud 'Om'. Keep holding the 'mmm' until the end of your breath. Repeat for 3–5 minutes.	1 Beginner, find which meditation type works for you. Then practise for 15 minutes once or twice a week. 2 Advanced – work up to 15 minutes of daily meditation.
Inner Peace/ nature	Go outside and re-connect with nature. Sit on grass or supported by a tree. Close your eyes and focus on feeling the Universal Energy.	1 Connect with nature twice a week. 2 Connect with nature daily.
Positive self-talk	Stop at various intervals during the day and assess whether your thoughts are positive or negative.	Consciously turn your negative thoughts into positive ones.
Positive Affirmations	Look at yourself in the mirror and repeat: I am wonderful. I am unique. I am enough.	Write down 3 positive affirmations and repeat them 3 times a day for 30 days.
Attitude of Gratitude	Write down 3 things which you are grateful for today.	Buy yourself a gratitude journal and write down daily what you are thankful for.
Daily Wins	Write down at least 2 wins which you have achieved today.	Write down your daily wins at the end of each day for 30 days. Reflect how you feel.
Friends and Family	Think of the best times in your life. Were you alone or who were you with? What made those times so amazing?	Decide if you have enough friends and family time allocated. Add in more phone calls and get togethers.
Calm Thinking	Think of something you need to think through. Set an alarm for 15–20 minutes. Talk the topic through out loud to yourself.	1 Find yourself a thinking friend and try the thinking technique. 2 locate yourself a quiet spot in nature where you can go to think.

Simply Well-Being

Appendix Two

Summary of all exercises and suggested actions for mental and physical well-being strategies.

PHYSICAL WELL-BEING STRATEGIES

	Try This Exercise	Suggested Action
Nutrition	Assess your current diet. Keep a food diary for a few weeks and record how you feel after each meal. Identify any food groups which do not make you feel good.	Keep a food diary. Add another vegetarian or vegan or fish dish to your week. Commit to your 5 a day for 30 days. Just one sweet snack per day. Eat breakfast daily.
Hydration	Write down what liquids you have consumed today. How many glasses of water do you typically have in one day?	Increase your daily water intake – this will depend on how much you drink currently.
Gut Health		Keep a diary of how you feel after eating. Do you feel bloated at all? Take a recommended pro/prebiotic and digestive enzyme daily for 30 days and reflect how you feel.
Skin Products	Write down all of the products which you use on your body daily.	Audit what products you use. Do they contain any harmful ingredients? Swap 1 or 2 of your daily products to a healthier brand.
Exercise		Decide on your exercise goal and write it down. Identify a form of exercise that you enjoy and schedule it into your diary. Examples – 15 minutes of movement daily, 10,000 steps, taking the stairs and no lifts, adding a mindfulness practise once a week.
Rest		Keep a sleep diary then assess any changes you need. Examples – commit to an extra 30 or 60 minutes of sleep a day, don't set an alarm once a week, exercise regularly, new nighttime routine, switch off technology an hour before bed, no caffeine after 5pm, meditating.

Acknowledgements

I've had this goal of writing and publishing a book for many years. Mainly because books have helped me so much throughout my life and, for me personal development is an ongoing journey. I hope to have contributed to the plethora of wisdom which is available via the written word.

There are many people I would like to thank, who have helped to make this dream a reality. Thank you firstly to my mum and dad who have supported me unconditionally throughout my life and who were the signposts for the start of my spiritual journey. I chose well when choosing you both as my parents. To my husband Gavin who hasn't a clue what this book is about, but who gave me the opportunity and time to get my thoughts down on paper when we moved our family to Switzerland. To all of my family and friends who have shared some of my life journey with me and helped me through the ups and downs. To those who have helped me shape and edit this book at various stages, your feedback, insight and encouragement have been invaluable, Sally van Gessel, Anne Ellsworth, Cecily Carmona and Paul Roberts.

And finally to you the reader, thank you for choosing my book.

About the Author

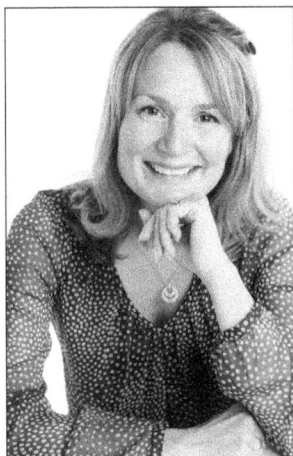

Mary Parrish is from the UK and, at the time of writing this book, lives in Switzerland with her husband and two children. She spent over 20 years of her life in Corporate Marketing and Project roles as well as training in alternative therapies in her spare time. She was able to pursue her love of well-being after the move to Switzerland when she finally had time to put pen to paper and get her thoughts down in this book. She is currently a business and well-being coach.

"Your Health is your Wealth" is her favourite motto!

Qualifications

Hypnotherapist

Spiritual Response Therapist

Reiki Healer

Energy Healer

Indian Head Massage Therapist

HypnoBirthing Practitioner

www.simply-well-being.com

Ingram Content Group UK Ltd.
Milton Keynes UK
UKHW020033160323
418612UK00015B/555